BACK PAIN AND OSTEOPOROSIS

Lee H. Riley III, M.D.,

and

Suzanne M. Jan de Beur, M.D.

JOHNS HOPKINS
MEDICINE

Dear Reader:

Welcome to the 2010 *Back Pain and Osteoporosis White Paper*—your personal guide to the prevention, diagnosis, and management of back pain and osteoporosis.

This year's highlights include:

- The link between **cardiovascular disease** and **low back pain**. (page 5)
- **Aquatic exercises** that **ease** low back pain. (page 12)
- **Injections** for **low back pain**: What you should know. (page 28)
- What to do when **back surgery fails**. (page 34)
- Which **vertebral compression fracture treatment** may be **no better than no treatment** at all? (page 37)
- Suffering from **back or neck pain**? Ask for an **exercise prescription**. (page 43)
- **Osteoporosis** and **diabetes**: A dangerous duo. (page 50)
- Can a **simple blood test** identify people at risk for **osteoporosis**? (page 56)
- A **three-pronged exercise plan** to protect yourself from **osteoporosis**. (page 60)
- Taking a **bisphosphonate** for osteoporosis? **Persistence** counts. (page 65)

If you have any back pain- or osteoporosis-related queries that you would like answered in the White Papers or comments about the White Papers in general, please e-mail the editors at whitepapers@johnshopkinshealthalerts.com.

Wishing you the best of health in 2010,

Lee H. Riley III, M.D.
Chief, Orthopedic Spine Division
Johns Hopkins Medicine

Suzanne M. Jan de Beur, M.D.
Director of Endocrinology
Johns Hopkins Bayview Medical Center

P.S. Please visit www.HopkinsBackPain.com for the latest news on back pain and osteoporosis and other information that will complement your Johns Hopkins White Paper.

MEDICAL EDITORS

Lee H. Riley III, M.D., received his M.D. from the Johns Hopkins University School of Medicine. He completed his residency in orthopedic surgery at Johns Hopkins and was a fellow in spine surgery at the University of Miami. He is an Associate Professor of Orthopedic Surgery and Neurosurgery and Chief of the Orthopedic Spine Division at Johns Hopkins Medicine.

■ ■ ■

Suzanne M. Jan de Beur, M.D., received her M.D. from Weill Medical College of Cornell University in New York City. She completed her internal medicine residency at Johns Hopkins Hospital and was an endocrinology fellow at Hopkins. Currently, she is Director of Endocrinology at Johns Hopkins Bayview Medical Center and an Associate Professor of Medicine at the Johns Hopkins University School of Medicine. She has special clinical expertise in metabolic bone disease and brings this clinical perspective to her laboratory research on molecular determinants of osteomalacia, disorders of phosphate homeostasis, and parathyroid hormone resistance syndromes. She has published extensively in leading journals, including *The New England Journal of Medicine, The Lancet,* and the *Journal of Bone and Mineral Research.*

CONTENTS

BACK PAIN

Four out of five adults experience significant low back pain at some point in their lives. This figure is not surprising, given the amount of stress placed on the back throughout the day. It not only supports the weight of the body during standing, walking, and lifting, but also turns, twists, and bends. These movements are affected by the strength, flexibility, and alignment of many body parts. As a result, seemingly simple movements—how we habitually stand or sit, for instance—can adversely affect our backs, sometimes to the point of injury.

This White Paper describes the major causes of back pain in adults, including:

- sprains, strains, and spasms
- degenerative changes of the spinal bones and disks
- herniated disks
- vertebral compression fractures
- spinal stenosis
- spinal deformities.

Also discussed are sciatica and cauda equina syndrome, two conditions caused by spinal stenosis or disk herniation.

Anatomy of the Spine

At birth, the human spine is composed of 33 interlocking bones, called vertebrae, which stack upon each other at a slight angle to form the spine's S-shaped curve. This distinctive curvature helps the spine act as a shock absorber when we move while still supporting the body's weight. The vertebrae grow progressively larger and stronger from top to bottom, and by adulthood, most people have only 24 vertebrae because some fuse together.

The seven delicate cervical (neck) vertebrae support the head; the larger 12 thoracic (chest) vertebrae bear the weight of the arms and trunk; and the five thickest and sturdiest lumbar (lower back) vertebrae carry the weight of the entire body (see the illustration on page 3). Because the lumbar region endures the greatest stress, it is the most vulnerable to strain or other problems. At the base of the spine are nine fused vertebrae that make up the sacrum (the back wall of the pelvis) and coccyx (tailbone). Each vertebra consists of a large oval block of bone (the vertebral body), pedicles, and lamina that surround the canal that the nerves run through, facets that articulate with the vertebrae above and below, two transverse bony projections (processes) that are points of attachment of spinal muscles, and a single spinous process that provides attachments for the muscles, ligaments, and tendons that connect one vertebra to another.

Between each vertebral body and the next is a flexible pad of cartilage-like tissue. This pad, which is called an intervertebral disk, cushions the vertebrae as the body moves. The high water content of the disks makes them very elastic—as we bend, twist, and move, they can expand, contract, and then return to their original shape. Thus, the disks, working in conjunction with the interlocking facet joints, give the spine its tremendous flexibility.

Yet another crucial function of the spine is to form a protective shell around the delicate spinal cord. At the rear of each vertebral body is a hole; when the vertebrae are stacked upon each other, these holes create a channel known as the spinal canal, through which the spinal cord runs. Spinal nerves, which branch off from the spinal cord through spaces (foramina) between adjacent vertebrae, extend to all parts of the body. The spinal cord ends at about waist level, dividing into a bundle of nerves that continues downward—the cauda equina (Latin for horse's tail, since its structure resembles the tail of a horse). Because of this intricate interweaving of bone and nerve tissue, problems with the vertebrae can cause symptoms from pressure on the spinal nerves or the spinal cord.

Causes of Back Pain

Most of the time, the exact cause of back pain is not easily determined. Fortunately, about 90% of cases improve on their own.

People under age 60 generally have acute backaches—that is, backaches that are sudden and short lived. These most often occur as pain limited to the back and result from a sprain or strain (it can be hard to distinguish between the two), a spasm, or, less frequently, a degenerated or herniated disk. In older people, chronic conditions such as degenerative changes of the spinal bones and disks, vertebral compression fractures, spinal stenosis (narrowing of the spinal column), and spinal deformities are the most common sources of back pain.

Other back-related disorders may cause symptoms that are not limited to back pain. For example, sciatica—pain that radiates into

The Aging Spine

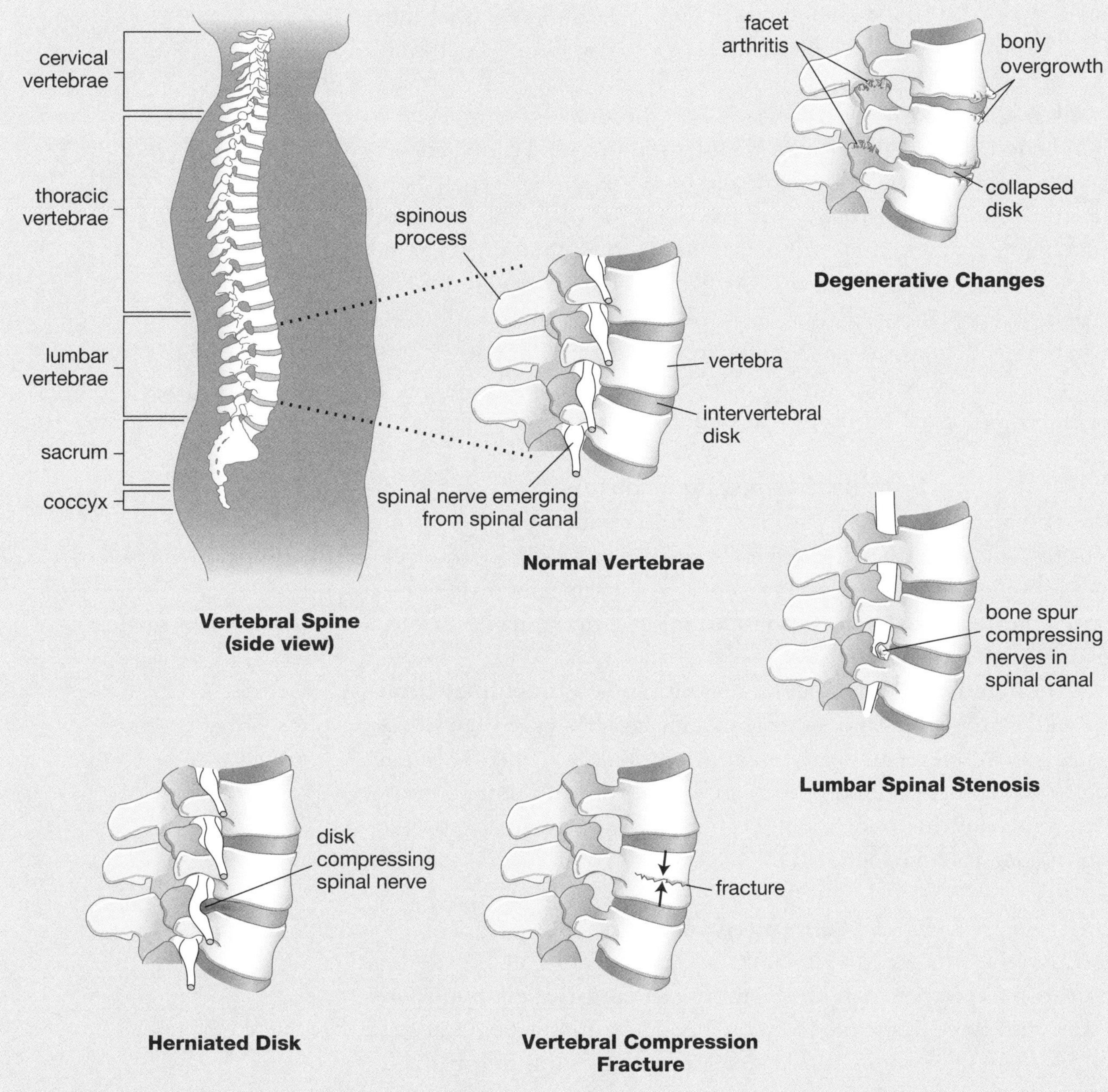

In adults, 24 vertebrae stacked together form the S-shaped spinal column, which supports the body's weight, allows for a wide range of movement, and ensheathes the delicate spinal cord. (The major parts of the spine, described in detail on pages 1-2, are illustrated above.)

As we age, the spine grows susceptible to injury and strain—especially in the lumbar region, which takes on most of the back's weight-bearing tasks. Also illustrated above are the four most common causes of back pain in older adults: degenerative changes (see page 4), herniated disk (see page 5), vertebral compression fractures (see page 6), and spinal stenosis (see page 7). ■

the buttocks, down the thighs to below the knees, and into the calves and often even the feet—is caused by irritation of a nerve leaving the spinal canal (the hollow channel through which the spinal cord runs) in the lumbar region of the back. Stiffness and loss of muscle strength may accompany back pain.

Although it may seem that back pain occurs suddenly (such as when bending down to pick up something), underlying problems—including normal aging, a weak back and weak abdominal muscles, obesity, and postural imbalances—set the stage for such "back attacks." The frequency of sprains and strains tends to decline after age 60, in part because older adults are less likely to participate in the kind of vigorous activities that lead to these problems. In addition, the disks between the vertebrae become less pliable in older adults and, as a result, are more likely to herniate. Such rigidity also may lead to degeneration of the various spinal bones.

Sprains, Strains, and Spasms

Sprains, strains, and spasms usually result from activity or injury. The term *sprain* is used when a ligament is partly torn, while *strain* applies to cases when a muscle is overstretched. A muscle spasm refers to a contraction of muscles in response to injury, which may occur in a ligament, muscle, disk, or joint.

Although the pain may be intense, muscle spasms ultimately protect you. Pain is your body's way of making sure that the injured area remains immobile, thus preventing further damage. Unlike back pain due to the compression of a nerve, the presence of a muscle spasm cannot be confirmed by imaging technology such as an x-ray or magnetic resonance imaging (MRI).

Degenerative Changes

Degenerative changes to the disks and facet joints in the lumbar spine, often referred to as degenerative osteoarthritis or spondylosis, are an inevitable consequence of aging. They usually begin around age 20, but imaging studies have detected changes within the disks of teenagers. Degenerative changes, along with vertebral compression fractures (see page 6) and kyphosis (see page 8), are responsible for the loss of height experienced by many people over age 50.

As we age, lumbar disks wear out because they are subjected to such large loads. Depending on what you do for a living and what types of activity you engage in during your leisure time, pressure on the lumbar spine can range from one to 11 times your body weight. Standing erect places a load on a lumbar disk equivalent to your body weight; bending, twisting, and lifting increase the load in proportion to the activity and the amount of weight lifted. Age-related loss of strength in the back muscles—which normally bear about one third of the load on the spine—also increases the stress on the disks and facet joints.

Over the years, the center of the disk slowly loses its water content and shrinks. This flattening of the disks leads to a narrowing of the space between the vertebrae. Further, as a result of supporting heavy loads, the vertebrae may develop bone spurs (osteophytes) that can press on a spinal nerve and cause pain.

Another possible cause of pain is deterioration of the facet joints due to disk wear and vertebral changes. In addition, arthritic changes (caused by a gradual erosion of the cartilage that lines the facet joints of the spine) can lead to pain and impair the smooth and coordinated movement of the spine (see the illustration on page 3). Pain also can occur if the nerves in the outer portion of the disks themselves are irritated.

Disk Herniation

About 10% of people experience symptoms from a herniated disk at some point in their lives. Autopsy studies reveal, however, that most people actually had a herniated disk during their lifetime but never experienced any symptoms.

Over the years, the demand of supporting the body's weight causes the outer layer of the disk to weaken, become thinner, and develop microscopic tears. At the same time, the center of the disk slowly loses its water content, so that it becomes progressively drier. These changes make the disk susceptible to herniation (protrusion), in which mild trauma such as lifting an object or even sneezing causes the center of the disk to bulge through the weakened outer layer.

Symptoms usually occur when the protruding disk presses on one or more of the spinal nerves emerging from the spinal column (see the illustration on page 3). In some people, the disk presses on the spinal cord itself or on the cauda equina. This causes pain not only in the back, but also in the part of the body served by the compressed and inflamed nerve. In some cases, disk fragments may break free, a condition referred to as sequestration. Although any disk can herniate, about 90 to 95% of cases occur in the two lowest disks, which bear the greatest weight.

When a disk herniates, both the site and extent of the rupture determine the location and severity of the symptoms. For example, a herniated lumbar disk may cause pain, numbness, or weakness in

NEW RESEARCH

Atherosclerosis Linked to Disk Degeneration and Low Back Pain

People with atherosclerosis—a buildup of fatty plaques in the walls of blood vessels—are more likely to experience disk degeneration and low back pain, according to a new systematic review.

Researchers examined data from 25 studies on atherosclerosis and back problems. Postmortem studies found a link between disk degeneration and fatty lesions in the aorta, as well as a link between blocked arteries to the lower back and low back pain. Clinical studies linked calcium buildup in the aorta to low back pain and linked narrowing of the lumbar arteries to both disk degeneration and low back pain. Observational studies linked smoking and high cholesterol levels to disk degeneration and low back pain.

Atherosclerosis can obstruct blood flow to the arteries that feed the spine. Could this diminished blood flow explain the higher rate of back problems? This study doesn't resolve whether the relationship is cause and effect; it's possible that underlying factors simply make some people more likely to develop both conditions.

Whether or not it can help your back, keeping your cardiovascular system in good condition is essential. That means maintaining a healthy lifestyle that includes smart eating habits, adequate exercise, and no smoking.

THE EUROPEAN JOURNAL OF VASCULAR AND ENDOVASCULAR SURGERY
Volume 37, page 661
February 17, 2009

one leg (sciatica). However, a herniated cervical disk may produce similar symptoms in one arm or hand (less commonly, both sides can be affected).

In general, a spasm of the back muscles plus difficulty walking or standing straight indicate a herniated disk; the spasm creates a recognizable leaning to one side in about half of those affected.

Pain due to a herniated disk usually strikes suddenly. The person may "feel something snap" before the pain begins—and the pain may start as a mild tingling or a "pins and needles" sensation before increasing in severity. If the herniated disk compresses the sciatic nerve, pain later radiates into a specific area of one leg. A decrease in back pain may be accompanied by increasingly severe pain, numbness, and weakness in one leg, along with changes in reflexes. In fact, a herniated lumbar disk is the most common cause of sciatica.

If a ruptured disk compresses nerves in the neck, pain may radiate down the arms and be accompanied by weakness and numbness in the arms and hands.

Vertebral Compression Fractures

A healthy vertebra will not break unless it is subjected to a forceful injury, such as that occurring in a car accident. In comparison, even minor trauma—such as a sneeze—can cause a compression fracture of a vertebra (see the illustration on page 3) that has been weakened by other conditions, such as:

- Osteoporosis (reduced bone mass), the most common cause of vertebral compression fractures. (Vertebral compression fractures related to osteoporosis are discussed in greater detail in the osteoporosis section; see pages 48-49 and 72-73.)
- Paget's disease, which is most common in older individuals. It is characterized by excessive breakdown of bone and the formation of weaker, disordered bone, especially in the spine, pelvis, skull, and femur (thighbone). This unorganized bone is weak and prone to fracture, although the condition may produce no symptoms.
- Hyperparathyroidism, which can also cause bone problems. People with hyperparathyroidism have a benign tumor of the parathyroid gland that produces excessive amounts of parathyroid hormone, which weakens bones by stimulating osteoclasts, the cells that break down bones, and by promoting the loss of calcium from bone.
- Cancer. Vertebral compression fractures, although rarely a first sign of cancer, can occur in people with cancer that has spread to the spine. This spread occurs most often with breast cancer, prostate cancer, and multiple myeloma.

Spinal Stenosis

Spinal stenosis—a narrowing of the spinal canal—is usually the result of degenerative changes in the spine, or it may develop as a complication of surgery, trauma to the spine, or involvement of the spine in Paget's disease. It typically affects people in their 50s and 60s.

As the body ages, gradual deterioration of the disks and facet joints in the spine causes the bones to rub together. This increased friction may eventually lead to the formation of overgrowths or bone spurs (called osteophytes) at the facet joints and around the rims of the vertebrae.

Spinal stenosis can occur when these overgrowths of bone gradually narrow the central canal of the spine; ligaments may thicken and cause narrowing of the spinal canal as well. The narrowing leads to symptoms as the spinal cord or the cauda equina becomes compressed (see the illustration on page 3). Symptoms can vary, ranging from vague numbness and weakness in the legs while standing and walking to severe pain and difficulties with bowel and bladder control.

Symptoms of spinal stenosis usually start slowly and are mild at first. Central stenosis can cause back pain, but usually the pain radiates into both legs. The pain does not follow the distribution of specific nerves but rather seems to involve the buttocks, thighs, calves, and, occasionally, the entire length of both legs.

The pain feels like cramping and may be associated with weakness, a "rubbery" feeling, numbness, and a sensation of loss of power in the legs. As a result of this weakness, people are prone to falls. Because the nerves controlling the bladder emerge from the lower spine, spinal stenosis may also cause urinary incontinence.

Vascular Claudication

The pain of spinal stenosis may be confused with that of another condition known as vascular claudication. This condition produces a cramping pain in the buttocks, thighs, or calves caused by impaired blood flow to the legs due to atherosclerosis (hardening of the arteries). However, the two conditions can be distinguished from each other by the pattern of the pain.

Pain due to vascular claudication stops quickly when you rest, even in the standing position. By comparison, pain due to spinal stenosis is related to body position and may continue for as long as you remain standing. Bending forward or sitting down usually relieves the pain, but even then the pain of spinal stenosis does not stop as quickly as pain resulting from insufficient blood flow.

Another tip for telling the two conditions apart: Individuals with vascular claudication have pain that starts in their feet or calves that radiates up toward their back and buttock, whereas people with spinal stenosis have pain that starts in their back and buttock and radiates down toward their feet.

Bed rest may increase spinal stenosis pain by exaggerating the natural curve of the lower back, which puts more pressure on the spinal nerves. A person with spinal stenosis may feel more comfortable when sitting in a forward-leaning position, which flexes the lower spine and relieves some of the pressure on the nerves. Likewise, when people with spinal stenosis stand, they may be more comfortable leaning slightly forward. Many people with spinal stenosis find that they tend to lean forward on a shopping cart while buying groceries. As the condition worsens, pain may occur while sitting, or it may wake the person at night.

Spinal Deformities

The two basic types of spinal deformities are kyphosis and scoliosis. These conditions usually develop during childhood or adolescence and worsen over time. However, they may develop in older people solely as the result of degenerative changes that occur with age.

Kyphosis

This condition is characterized by extensive flexion (bending forward) of the spine. It usually affects the upper back (the thoracic spine) but may also occur in the neck or lower back. Thoracic kyphosis is sometimes referred to as dowager's hump, humpback, or hunchback. Kyphosis is particularly common in older women and can result from disk degeneration (in which the disks lose moisture and shrink), vertebral fractures due to osteoporosis, or both.

Severe thoracic kyphosis reduces the amount of space available for the lungs and other organs, potentially leading to breathing problems or a protruding abdomen. It can also lead to difficulty finding clothes that fit properly.

Scoliosis

Defined as an abnormal sideways bend to the back, scoliosis is caused by a twisting of the spine. It can occur at any location in the spine. The amount of pain caused by scoliosis usually depends on the degree of the deformity; more pronounced bends tend to be more painful. Most scoliosis in our society develops in childhood; however, it may progress later in life because of disk degeneration.

Scoliosis occurring from degenerative changes alone tends to create fewer problems than childhood scoliosis.

Sciatica and Cauda Equina Syndrome

Sciatica, which affects 40% of adults during their lifetime, can occur when lateral spinal stenosis or a herniated disk irritates some part of either sciatic nerve. Each large sciatic nerve is formed by nerve roots that emerge from the lower spine, join together in the hip region, and run down the back of each thigh. Near the knee, the sciatic nerves branch into smaller nerves that extend into the calves, ankles, feet, and toes.

Sciatica results from irritation of one of the nerve roots in the lower back, most often those emanating from the fourth lumbar vertebra (L4), fifth lumbar vertebra (L5), or first sacral vertebra (S1). Pain or numbness develops along the path of the sciatic nerve; the precise location of symptoms depends on which spinal nerve root is affected. Compression of the sciatic nerves can also diminish leg strength.

After age 50, sciatica is more commonly caused by spinal stenosis than disk herniation. Most of the time, sciatica from a herniated disk resolves within six weeks with little or no treatment. In up to 50% of cases, sciatica from spinal stenosis resolves by itself within a month, but 25% may have pain for as long as four months.

Compression of the cauda equina may result in the sudden onset of impaired bowel and bladder function (usually an inability to empty the bowel or bladder or, conversely, incontinence); loss of sensation in the groin, buttocks, and legs; and severe weakness or paralysis in the legs. These symptoms—known as cauda equina syndrome—indicate an emergency situation that requires immediate surgical attention. People who cannot reach their doctor quickly should go to the emergency room of a nearby hospital for treatment.

Sciatica or cauda equina syndrome is usually due to one of the major disorders of the spine, such as disk herniation, degenerative changes of the spinal disks, spinal stenosis, or vertebral fracture.

Additional Causes of Back Pain

Other medical conditions that affect the spine and can lead to back pain include ankylosing spondylitis, osteomalacia, spondylolysis, spondylolisthesis, and vertebral osteomyelitis.

Ankylosing spondylitis

This condition is a chronic inflammation of the facet joints and the joints located between the back wall of the pelvis and the hip (the sacroiliac joints). Inflammation may also involve locations where ligaments and tendons attach to bone. In severe cases, the vertebrae may become fused together, resulting in rigidity and a stooped posture.

Osteomalacia

Bone is mostly composed of collagen but requires the minerals calcium and phosphorus for strength. Osteomalacia develops when the bones soften because of a lack of these minerals.

The most common cause of osteomalacia is vitamin D deficiency. Many older people suffer from a vitamin D deficiency. Vitamin D is essential for absorption of calcium and phosphorus (for more information, see the section on Vitamin D, beginning on page 59). Fractures due to osteomalacia are more common in the pelvis and ribs but may also involve the spine.

Spondylolysis

Spondylolysis is a defect and weakness in a portion of the spine called the pars interarticularis, a small segment of bone joining the facet joints in the back of the spine. The condition is basically a stress fracture in the pars interarticularis and is either congenital (present at birth) or may be caused later in life by trauma.

Spondylolisthesis

Spondylolisthesis, in which one of the vertebrae slips forward onto an adjacent vertebra, causes a gradual deformity of the lower spine and narrowing of the vertebral canal. It may develop in people with spondylolysis (see above), can be congenital, or may develop later in life because of disk degeneration associated with abnormal facet joints.

Vertebral osteomyelitis

This disorder is a serious and increasingly common bacterial infection of the spine that causes pain in the neck or back and may or may not be accompanied by fever. It is often associated with autoimmune disorders such as type 1 diabetes (which is sometimes called juvenile or insulin-dependent diabetes).

Cancer

In rare instances, back pain is caused by cancer in the spine. Malignant tumors of the spine account for far less than 1% of all cases of back pain and occur more frequently in older people. Cancer can originate in the vertebrae, as in the case of multiple myeloma (cancer cells that move from the bone marrow to the bones at numerous sites). It can also spread to the spine from other sites in the body, most often from the breast, prostate, lung, kidney, or thyroid gland.

Other causes

Not all back pain is caused by problems with the spine or back muscles. In some cases, pain originates in the abdominal organs and radiates to the back. Conditions such as pancreatitis (inflammation of the pancreas), peptic ulcers (lesions in the stomach or small intestine), or an abdominal aortic aneurysm (a ballooning of the wall of the body's largest artery, which carries blood from the heart to the rest of the body) may also cause back pain.

In addition, back pain may originate from gallstones, kidney stones, kidney infections, and endometriosis (a growth of the tissue lining a woman's uterus in places other than the uterus). Last, but certainly not least, emotional stress may induce back pain.

Diagnosing Back Pain

After the common cold, back pain is the problem that most frequently brings people to a doctor's office. It is often difficult to pinpoint the exact cause of back pain because so many different body structures can be involved.

Fortunately, most episodes of back pain—about 90%—will clear up with little or no treatment in approximately six weeks, reducing the need for medical intervention. As long as you are not experiencing severe back pain or other symptoms (such as severe nighttime pain or pain that worsens with lying down, weight loss, bowel or bladder dysfunction, or fever) that might indicate a serious health condition such as cancer, infection, cauda equina syndrome, or an abdominal aortic aneurysm, you can safely try self-treatment (see pages 24-25).

Back pain due to muscle injury typically subsides completely in about six to eight weeks. Back pain that lasts longer than this is usually due to spinal column changes and merits a visit to a physician.

Signs and Symptoms

Few back pain episodes require immediate medical treatment. However, to rule out the possibility of a dangerous condition, doctors still need to ask certain questions routinely—for example, whether you can relieve the pain by changing your position and whether you feel pain when you're not moving.

Working Out in Water

Try aquatic exercise to help manage low back pain

The health benefits of water therapy have been acknowledged throughout history. Many ancient civilizations, like those of the Greeks, Romans, and Chinese, recognized the natural healing properties of water, and they used it to help treat various ailments, including muscle pain. Today, we also use water therapy (otherwise known as hydrotherapy or aquatic therapy) to manage various musculoskeletal conditions, including low back pain.

How Does Water Therapy Help?

We all know that water benefits us from the "inside out"— hence the oft cited advice to drink eight glasses of water each day. Water also provides numerous benefits from the "outside in." For instance, working out in water can increase your cardiovascular fitness, improve your flexibility, and help you relax. If you have back problems, aquatic exercise can also help to:

Stabilize your lower back. Water naturally resists when you move. Exercising against this resistance, with the right pushing or pulling motions, gently develops muscle strength in your back, abdomen, and hips. When you target these core muscles, you help stabilize your posture and support your lower back. The deeper you immerse your body, the greater the resistance and the more challenging the water workout will be.

Minimize pressure on your spine, joints, and muscles. Because water is buoyant, it supports your weight, thereby minimizing the pressure placed on your spine, joints, and muscles. This results in a number of benefits. First, the reduced stress can help alleviate pain and decrease the chances of further aggravating your back. Second, you can move through the water with relative ease, which enables you to stretch your back muscles and improve your range of motion.

Third, you're able to perform movements in water that may be too difficult or painful to carry out on a hard surface during land-based exercises.

Soothe and relax your muscles. Even without exercising, being in warm water—as is generally recommended for people recovering from a back injury—can relieve pain, reduce swelling, and relax your back muscles. In addition, the soothing, warm water environment may motivate you to exercise more consistently and, in turn, enable you to achieve better results from your exercise routine.

Getting Started Safely

If you're considering getting into the pool, Kelly Daley, senior P.T. at John's Hopkins Hospital's Department of Physical Medicine and Rehabilitation, offers the following advice.

If you're recovering from a back injury, it's probably best to meet with a physical therapist who can design a safe aquatic exercise routine that incorporates warm-water stretches to relieve pain and improve range of motion. You'll also learn how to keep your spine properly aligned in the water.

Most water workouts should be done while submerged in warm water that is chest to waist deep. The deeper you are, the greater the water's buoyancy and cushioning. If you have a severe back injury, you may need to begin exercising while submerged to the neck (assisted by flotation devices). This position reduces pressure on the spinal nerves and soft tissues and decreases pain. As your spine grows stronger and is able to tolerate partial weight-bearing exercise, you'll make a transition to more shallow water.

If you're not able to work with a physical therapist, you may want to try some of the following aquatic exercises. Be sure to get your doctor's okay first.

Each exercise strengthens specific areas of the back, so depending on the source of your pain, some exercises may be more beneficial than others. Begin with the number of repetitions suggested (if you are able) and slowly increase to double the repetitions. ■

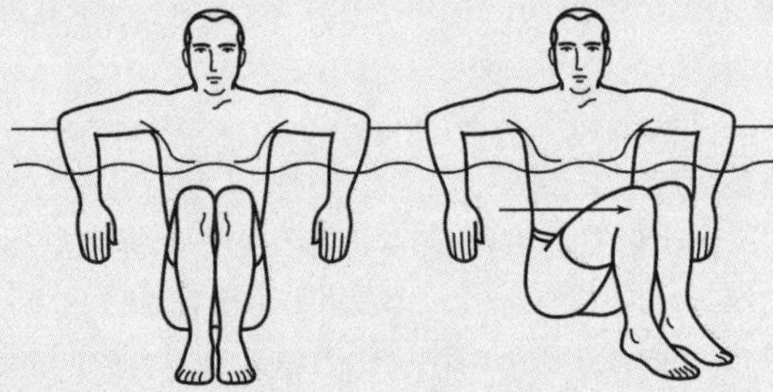

Lumbar Rotation

- Prop arms up on pool ledge with your back to the wall.
- Bend your knees, bringing them to your chest.
- Tighten your abdominals.
- Rotate legs from left to right.
- Return legs to the center and straighten them, with your feet down.
- Perform 2 sets of 5 repetitions.

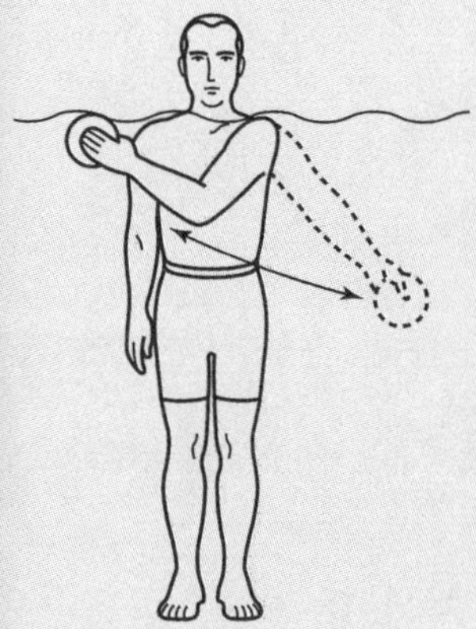

Shoulder Diagonal I
- Stand in shoulder-height water with left arm out at 45-degree angle.
- In left hand, hold drag device (a mitt-like device that provides resistance and is available at sporting goods stores).
- Tighten your abdominal muscles.
- Move left arm up and inward across body, toward the surface of the water. (Bending elbow slightly during movement is fine.)
- Return to start position and repeat. Perform 2 sets of 10 repetitions.
- Repeat with right arm.

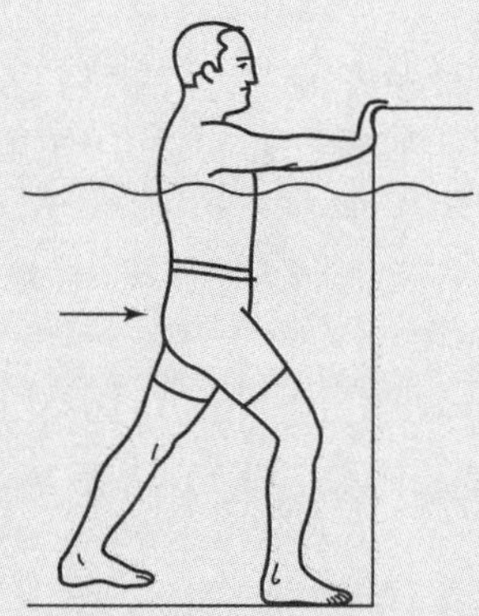

Calf Stretch
- Stand in chest-high water facing pool wall, hands on the ledge.
- Without arching your back, step forward with right foot, leaning hips toward wall.
- Keep left leg straight with heel on the pool bottom.
- Hold the stretch for 20 to 30 seconds.
- Perform the stretch twice with each leg.

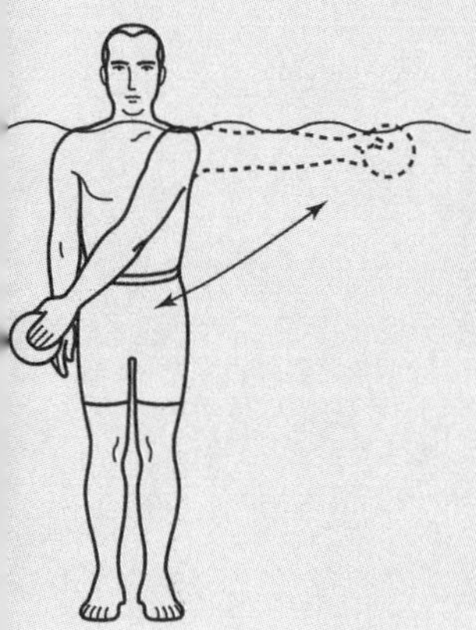

Shoulder Diagonal II
- Stand in shoulder-height water with left arm across body at opposite hip.
- Hold drag device in left hand.
- Tighten your abdominal muscles.
- Move left arm up and outward away from body, toward the surface of the water. (Bending elbow slightly during movement is fine.)
- Return to start position and repeat. Perform 2 sets of 10 repetitions.
- Repeat with right arm.

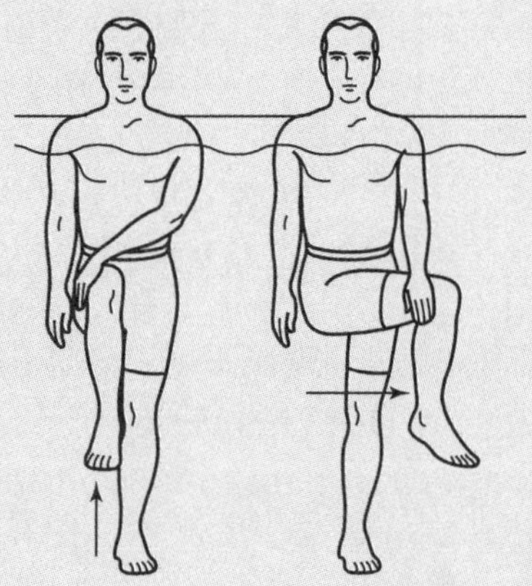

Gluteal Stretch
- Stand in chest-high water with back to pool wall.
- Without arching or twisting your back, bring your right knee up to your chest and grasp with the opposite hand.
- Rotate right thigh inward while pulling across chest.
- Hold the stretch for 20 to 30 seconds.
- Perform the stretch twice with each leg.

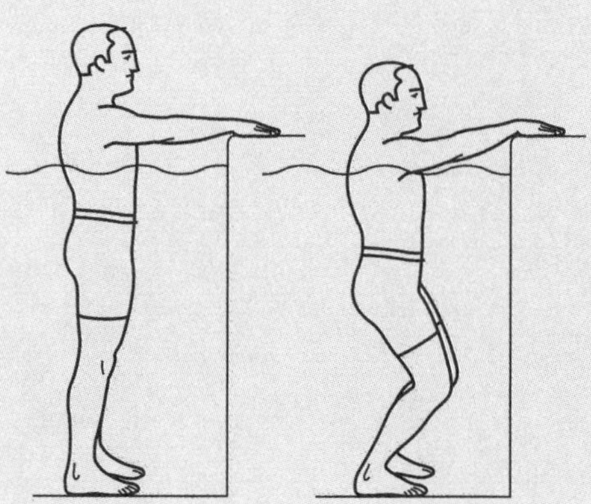

Knee Squat
- Stand in chest-high water, feet shoulder-width apart.
- Tighten your abdominals.
- Slowly squat down, keeping heels on the pool bottom.
- Stand back up.
- Do 2 sets of 5 repetitions.

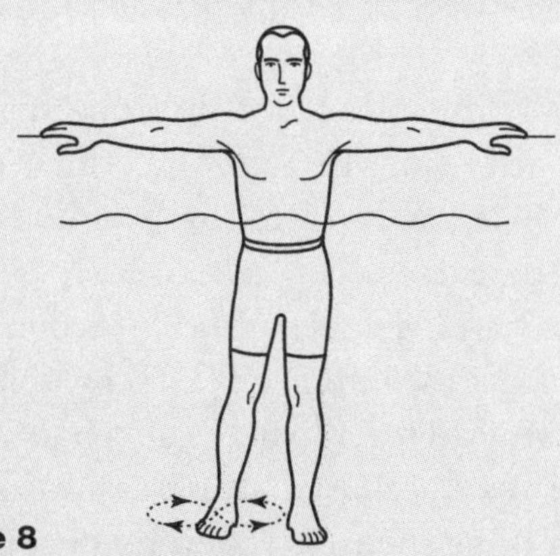

Hip Figure 8
- Stand in waist-deep water with your back to the pool wall.
- Place arms out to side on pool ledge.
- Tighten your abdominal muscles.
- Keep left knee straight and move right leg in a clockwise figure-8 motion.
- Reverse the motion in a counterclockwise direction.
- Repeat with left leg.
- Perform 2 sets of 5 repetitions for each leg.

Illustrations by Susan Blubaugh

Back Pain History

Some of the best clues to the cause of your back pain will come from your description of the pain. Obtaining an accurate account is a doctor's primary method of tracking down the cause and determining whether and what type of treatment is necessary. Questions your doctor will ask include:

• Where is the pain located? Is it confined to the lower back or does it radiate to the buttocks or legs? (These questions check for sciatica.)

• How severe is the pain? For example, is the pain so excruciating that any movement is difficult or impossible? Can you go about your normal daily activities, even though the pain prevents vigorous exercise or activities associated with a lot of bending and twisting, such as gardening or golf? (A good description of pain intensity can help the doctor determine its cause.)

• When did the pain begin? Was it related to an activity or an injury? (If the pain follows an injury, it is less likely to be due to a slowly progressing condition, such as spinal stenosis.)

• What makes your back feel better or worse? For example, does lying down make it feel better? Does bending forward to tie a shoe increase the pain? (The pattern of pain may indicate whether a nerve is involved, possibly because of a disk herniation.)

• Have you had a prior episode of back pain? If so, how was it treated and how effective was the treatment? (The condition may have recurred.)

• Do you have any other health problems? (Weight loss and poor appetite, for example, raise the concern that cancer has spread to the vertebrae. In addition, some disorders, such as hyperthyroidism, can cause osteoporosis.)

• What medications do you take? (Certain drugs, such as corticosteroids or anticonvulsants, can affect spinal bone mass.)

• What do you do for a living, and what kinds of exercise or other activities do you do? In what ways is the pain disabling? (Muscle injury is frequently related to a particular activity.)

Physical Examination

During a physical exam, your doctor will typically focus on your back, legs, and feet. The doctor will look at your posture and curvature of the spine; a hands-on examination of areas that are sore may provide clues to the origin of the pain. To observe muscles and joints during movement, the doctor may ask you to sit, stand, walk (including on your toes or heels), twist, or bend forward or sideways.

A neurological exam, including tests of sensation, strength, and reflexes, will be conducted as well. These tests are important to detect disorders such as disk herniation and spinal stenosis, as the nerves emerging from each level of the spine are responsible for sensation and muscle strength in specific parts of the body.

For example, the nerve issuing from underneath the fifth lumbar vertebra (L5) is responsible for sensation in a narrow band that runs down the upper leg and wraps around to the front of the lower leg and the top of the foot. By detecting loss of sensation in a particular area or diminished strength in certain muscles, the doctor may be able to determine which level of the spine is causing the pain. Reduced reflexes at specific areas also can provide vital clues to the source of back pain.

Another important component of the physical examination is the straight-leg-raise test, which can help the doctor determine whether disk herniation is responsible for the pain. During this exam, you lie on your back while the physician lifts each leg separately without bending the knee. The test is positive if raising the leg produces the typical symptoms—pain or tingling below the knee. The straight-leg-raise test is also helpful in monitoring the progress of treatment once a diagnosis has been made. Last, a rectal examination may be done to assess the nerve function of the anus, because the nerves of the anus arise from the lower lumbar spine.

Laboratory Tests

Routine blood tests help determine the cause of back problems in a few situations. Results may reflect the presence of inflammation and/or an infection. For example:

- Blood levels of alkaline phosphatase (an enzyme released by bone-forming cells called osteoblasts) are often extremely high in people with active Paget's disease (which can cause vertebral compression fractures and spinal stenosis).
- Blood calcium levels are elevated in people with hyperparathyroidism (which, along with osteoporosis, can lead to vertebral compression fractures).
- Prostate-specific antigen (PSA), which is elevated in men with prostate cancer, can be measured by a blood test to determine whether back pain is due to the spread of prostate cancer.
- Abnormal proteins in blood and urine are often present in people with multiple myeloma (cancer of the plasma cells, a type of white blood cell).

Imaging Studies

Diagnostic imaging studies provide a view of the bones and the soft tissues, which comprise muscles, ligaments, cartilage, tendons, and blood vessels. These studies are usually done when surgery might be necessary, when the doctor suspects a serious condition may be responsible for the back pain, or when you are experiencing severe pain. Experts advise against routine imaging studies when no particular cause of the pain is identified through the physical examination, patient history, and laboratory tests. When imaging is ordered, the study chosen depends, in large part, on what is suspected to be causing the pain.

X-rays

For chronic pain and for new-onset back pain lasting longer than four to six weeks, x-rays should be the first imaging study. They are especially useful for detecting fractures and invasion of bone by multiple myeloma. Although x-rays tend to be overused, they are useful for people over age 50, because this age group has a greater risk of malignancy and vertebral fractures. Modern x-rays are low enough in radiation to be considered safe, but should be used only when necessary. Conventional x-rays are available almost anywhere and are relatively low in cost.

Computed tomography (CT) scans

During a CT scan, also called a computerized axial tomography (CAT) scan, a thin x-ray beam is rotated around a specific area of the body to create a cross-sectional picture. CT scans are 10 to 20 times more sensitive than x-rays; they provide better soft-tissue detail and good detail of the vertebrae. Although CT myelograms (see below) or magnetic resonance imaging (MRI) scans (see page 17) are even more useful for examining the soft tissues (for example, herniated disks), CT scans are still best for studying bone problems—for example, bone destruction due to infection. CT scans are considerably more expensive and deliver more radiation than conventional x-rays.

CT myelogram

This procedure combines a CT scan and a myelogram (also known as myelography), a diagnostic tool that uses contrast dye that is injected into the fluid of the spinal canal. The contrast dye illuminates the spinal canal, cord, and nerve roots during imaging. A CT scan is taken after the dye is injected; the images produced clearly show both the bony structures of the spine and the nerve structures. The injection carries the risk of infection and side effects such as nausea, headaches, and pain or discomfort at the site of injection. People are required to sit or lie with their head elevated for six to eight hours afterward. These scans offer the best detail of bone and soft tissue. CT myelograms are usually performed only prior to surgery or after failed surgery.

MRI

In MRI, a person is surrounded with a powerful magnet. The magnet causes atomic nuclei in the body to vibrate and give out characteristic signals, which are then converted into two- and three-dimensional images. No x-rays are involved. This test provides the clearest images of soft tissues and is completely safe. Despite its precision, studies have shown that MRI should be reserved for certain specific indications.

MRI may not generate a useful image of the bones in the spine. Therefore, it is not recommended for early diagnosis of back pain unless the doctor suspects a serious condition, such as cauda equina syndrome, sciatica, or spinal stenosis. Even when an MRI is warranted, some drawbacks must be considered.

First, the abnormalities revealed may not necessarily be the cause of the back pain. Second, because people must lie perfectly still for a long period (anywhere from 30 minutes to two hours) in a relatively small space, the procedure may be uncomfortable and difficult to tolerate, especially for people who are claustrophobic. (An open MRI produces less claustrophobia than a closed machine but generally does not provide high-quality views and is not recommended if you can tolerate a standard MRI scanner.)

In addition, MRI cannot be used in people with certain devices, such as implantable cardioverter-defibrillators, pacemakers, or aneurysm clips. If you have any of these devices or questions about the safety of an MRI scan in your case, it's best to speak with your doctor about it.

Bone scans

Bone scans measure the amount of radioactivity emitted from bone after an injection of a bone-seeking compound that contains technetium, a radioactive metal. The bone is scanned two to three hours after the injection, and information about the distribution of the radioactive compound in the bone is fed into a computer, which produces a one- or two-dimensional image of the bone.

An area of bone that displays an increased uptake of technetium

ASK THE DOCTOR

Q. ***When my mother had back pain, her doctor ordered an x-ray. When I went to see my own doctor about back pain, however, he said I didn't need one. Should I be worried that my doctor is trying to cut corners?***

A. Not at all. In fact, clinical guidelines first put out in 1994 say that the only people who need x-rays for new back pain are those who have "red flags" for a condition such as cancer, infection, or compression of the cauda equina (the nerve roots below the spinal cord).

A new study that analyzed data on approximately 1,800 patients from six randomized, controlled trials confirm this recommendation. The researchers, publishing their analysis in the journal *The Lancet*, found no significant short-term (up to three months) or long-term (six to12 months) advantage to immediate spinal imaging with regards to pain or physical function.

Some doctors persist in ordering an x-ray for everyone with back pain, perhaps to reassure themselves or their patients that all is well. But x-rays are costly and expose patients to radiation. More important, they're unable to help a doctor decide whether surgery is necessary.

The fact that your doctor didn't perform an x-ray is good news, because you clearly didn't have any red flags and you didn't undergo an unnecessary test.

has a higher rate of bone turnover, which can be the result of a fracture or nonunion not identified on an x-ray. It can also indicate the presence of metastatic cancer, Paget's disease, or osteomyelitis (a bacterial infection of the spine).

The amount of radiation delivered is similar to that of a CT scan. This technique can be used to identify fractures in both the central and peripheral areas of the body.

Electrical Tests

Three basic types of electrical tests may be used in difficult cases involving leg pain that has persisted for over a month. These tests may help the doctor pinpoint the source of pain or numbness or suggest the cause of pain (for example, whether it is due to disk herniation or nerve damage from an unrelated disorder, such as diabetes).

Electromyography. In this test, electrodes are used to measure muscle abnormalities.

Nerve conduction and sensory-evoked potentials. These two tests examine nerve function by measuring how fast the nerves conduct impulses.

All three of the electrical tests are used only when the diagnosis is in doubt. But there is still some debate over their usefulness.

Preventing Back Pain

Because back pain may recur, it is especially important for anyone with a history of back problems to take steps to reduce their risk of damage to the spine and related structures. Measures that can be used for prevention include paying close attention to posture and body mechanics (habitual ways of moving), stretching and strengthening particular muscles, changing daily routines to protect the back, and, if necessary, using special products to help reduce strain on the back.

Improving Posture

Contrary to popular belief, standing at attention like a military recruit—with the head and shoulders rigidly pulled back and the lower back excessively arched—is not correct posture and can actually be hard on the back. Good posture allows the body to follow the natural S-shaped curve of the spine. As simple as that sounds, however, poor habits, previous injuries, and even ill-fitting shoes can contribute to improper spinal alignment. Poor posture can strain muscles and ligaments and increase the risk of compressed nerves.

The easiest way to evaluate your posture is to stand sideways in front of a mirror when you're not wearing any bulky clothing. Ideally, it should be possible to visualize a vertical line running straight from the front of your earlobe through the front of your shoulder, down the center of your hip, just behind your kneecap, and just in front of your ankle bone. Your chin should be parallel to the floor, not thrust outward. Alternatively, stand with your heels against a wall. If the back of your head, shoulders, buttocks, and calves touch the wall—and you can slide your hand between the wall and your lower back—you have good alignment.

To check your posture while sitting, sit in an armless chair with your side to a mirror. You should be able to visualize a line running through the same points of your upper body down to the center of your hip. Perpetual slouching with the shoulders rolled forward causes kyphosis. Mild kyphosis (see page 8) can usually be corrected through a program of exercise. More severe cases may require surgical correction.

Posture varies with age. As people get older and lose height because of disk changes, the curve in the lumbar region of the back tends to straighten, leading to a slight stoop, which is normal. In addition, the curve in the thoracic region tends to become accentuated with age. The following tips will help to improve poor posture.

Standing

When standing, keep your head level and your chin slightly tucked in. Stand tall, stretching the top of your head towards the ceiling. Relax your shoulders and tighten your stomach muscles to tuck in your stomach.

Standing for long periods can be tiring and lead to bad posture. Distributing your weight so you are aligned vertically (a straight line from the point between your eyes to your chin, collarbone, breastbone, pelvis, and midpoint between your ankles) can relieve fatigue and maintain good posture.

Sitting and lying down

When sitting, use a straight-backed chair, and sit with your shoulders against the chair back, your chest lifted, your arms on the armrests, and your upper back straight. An ideal chair includes armrests to support the weight of your arms, thereby reducing the pressure on your back. Avoid low, soft chairs that are difficult to get into and out of. Your feet should comfortably touch the floor, with your knees positioned slightly higher than your hips. You may need to place a footstool or thick book underneath your feet. When sitting for any length of time, it is important to get up and move around every 30 minutes or so.

When driving, adjust your seat position so that your knees are slightly higher than your hips and in a position that you can comfortably reach the steering wheel, brakes, and accelerator. Shift your hand position on the steering wheel frequently to minimize stress on the muscles in the upper back and neck.

When in bed, lying on one side with knees bent and a pillow between them helps to maintain the natural curves of the spine. Place a pillow under your knees when sleeping on your back.

Exercising To Protect and Strengthen the Back

Regular exercise can help people lose excess weight and improve their overall health. It can also help prevent back pain and injury. A review of numerous studies focusing on exercise to protect the back found that people who worked out regularly experienced less back pain and had fewer sick days due to back pain than those who didn't exercise.

Exercises for back pain focus on strengthening the muscles in the back and abdomen and stretching the muscles in the back. Flexibility exercises for your hips and even your shoulders may also be needed, because improving your flexibility in these areas will decrease the demands on your back.

Ask your doctor to refer you to a physical therapist, who can instruct you in exercises such as the pelvic tilt, cat stretch, and "crunches" (partial sit-ups). Walking also is an effective way to strengthen the back and improve posture.

Avoiding Back Strain

In addition to correct posture and exercise, many other aspects of your daily life influence the health of your back. Some people simply need to improve the techniques that they use to perform everyday activities—lifting heavy objects, playing sports, or even getting in and out of a chair, for instance. Other people will need to avoid certain activities altogether.

Lift heavy objects properly

One study found that people who lifted objects improperly had twice the risk of a herniated disk as those who used the correct technique. To lift something safely, always bend at the knees and carry the object close to the body. The farther away from the body you hold an object, the more pressure is placed on your spine. Holding objects at arm's length can increase the load on the lower spine by 15 times the original weight. For example, when a person carries a 10-lb box at arm's length from the body, it is putting 150 lbs of pressure on the spine.

Choose activities wisely

Depending on the severity of your back problem, you may need to stay away from activities that require sudden twisting movements, including sports such as golf, bowling, football, basketball, baseball, weight lifting, and tennis and other racquet sports.

However, if your physician approves, you may be able to continue some of these activities as long as you modify your technique. In golf, for example, twisting movements during the swing must be minimized. In addition, golfers should keep their knees bent and spine straight when placing a ball on the tee or picking it up from the cup. Because improper serving and backhand techniques in tennis can strain the back, consider getting help with your technique from a tennis pro.

Maintain a healthy weight

Obesity places an extra burden on the lower back. It also increases the natural curve of the lumbar spine, forcing the vertebrae to bear weight at abnormal angles.

Quit smoking

Studies show that cigarette smoking decreases blood circulation in the intervertebral disks and speeds their degeneration. Smoking is also a major risk factor for osteoporosis.

Consider going to "back school"

Back schools are usually directed by a physical therapist, sometimes with the aid of a physician. They provide a safe, inexpensive, and effective way to learn more about how the back works and what can go wrong.

The school's director can analyze how your working conditions, daily activities, and even your sleeping habits may be harming your back. The school can customize an exercise program for you. Some schools also give instruction in relaxation techniques. A family doctor or physical therapist will have information about nearby schools.

Commonly Used Drugs for Relieving Back Pain 2010

Drug type: Brand (generic)	Typical daily dosages*	How to take	How they work
Analgesic			
Tylenol, other brands (acetaminophen)	1,300-6,000 mg	In several doses per day, with water.	May inhibit receptors that transmit pain signals. Does not reduce inflammation.
Nonsteroidal anti-inflammatory drugs (NSAIDs)			
Advil, Motrin IB (ibuprofen) (ketoprofen)† Aleve, Anaprox, Naprosyn (naproxen) Anacin, Bayer, other brands (aspirin) (diflunisal)† (meclofenamate)† Celebrex (celecoxib)	800-2,400 mg 200-225 mg 220-440 mg 1,950-3,900 mg 500-1,000 mg 200-400 mg 200-400 mg	*All except Celebrex:* Take with a full glass of water along with food, milk, or antacid. Limit alcohol while taking. Do not chew or crush pills. *Meclofenamate:* After taking, do not lie down for 30 minutes. *Celebrex:* Take with or without food.	Decrease inflammation and relieve pain by blocking prostaglandins, substances that induce pain, swelling, and fever.
Muscle relaxants			
Amrix, Flexeril (cyclobenzaprine) Robaxin (methocarbamol) Soma (carisoprodol)	15-30 mg 4,000-6,000 mg 1,050-1,400 mg	2-4x/day. Exactly as directed. 3x/day and at bedtime.	Relax skeletal muscle and relieve spasm without interfering with muscle action.
Anticonvulsant			
Neurontin (gabapentin)	1,200 mg (individualized)	With or without food.	Seems to decrease sensitivity of spinal nerves that transmit pain signals.
Antidepressants			
(amitriptyline)† Norpramin (desipramine)	50-150 mg 100-200 mg	4x/day; largest dose at bedtime.	Enhance levels of neurotransmitters (such as serotonin) in the brain that are believed to reduce pain sensations.
Opiates			
Avinza, Kadian, Oramorph SR (morphine) Darvon (propoxyphene) Demerol (meperidine) Dolophine, Methadose (methadone) Endocet, Percocet, Roxicet, Roxilox, Tylox (oxycodone/acetaminophen) Percodan (oxycodone/aspirin) Ultracet (tramadol/acetaminophen) Ryzolt, Ultram (tramadol) ***Long-acting:*** MS Contin (controlled-release morphine) OxyContin (controlled-release oxycodone)	40-180 mg 210-390 mg 300-1,200 mg 15-40 mg 4-6 tablets 4-6 tablets 4-8 tablets 50-300 mg 30-60 mg Highly individualized	*Percocet, Ultracet:* With food or milk. *Long-acting opiates:* Do not chew, break, or crush. This could cause a fatal overdose.	Depress the nervous system to inhibit perception of pain. *Percodan:* Also inhibits prostaglandins that cause inflammation. *Ultracet:* Also inhibits receptors that transmit pain signals.

Precautions	Most common side effects	Tell your doctor if...
Exceeding recommended dosage may cause liver or kidney damage, especially when combined with alcohol. Check with your doctor before taking any over-the-counter analgesic.	Fewer than most other drugs, except for rare allergic reactions (see symptoms at right).	You need to take it for more than 10 days. You have had ulcers or develop rash, hives, swelling, breathing difficulty.
May cause ulcers or internal bleeding. All drugs in this class (with the exception of aspirin) may increase the risk of heart attack and stroke. Avoid if you have asthma or liver, kidney, or heart problems. Check with your doctor before taking any over-the-counter NSAID.	Stomach irritation and many kinds of digestive problems (occur less with enteric-coated or buffered types); rash; itching, headache. Diflunisal may cause insomnia or drowsiness.	You develop rash, hives, swelling, difficulty breathing, vision problems, stomach cramps, heartburn, indigestion, you have had ulcers or internal bleeding in the past, you need to take the drug for more than 10 days.
Do not use if you have arrhythmia or heart failure. Use alcohol with caution. Drowsiness may interfere with driving and use of machinery. *Soma:* Has addictive potential. *Flexeril:* Should be used for no more than 2 or 3 weeks. Do not use if you take MAO inhibitors.	Drowsiness, dry mouth, dizziness, clumsiness, headache, rash, upset stomach, nausea, vomiting, blurred vision.	*Robaxin:* You have kidney or liver disease, vision or digestion changes, urinary problems, dizziness, sudden mood changes. *Flexeril or Soma:* You develop severe drowsiness, confusion, hallucinations, heart palpitations, seizures.
People over age 50 may need to take lower doses to avoid drug build up. May impair ability to use machinery. When ending treatment, taper off usage over 5-7 days.	Dizziness, vision problems, clumsiness, sleepiness, shaking or tremor, swelling of hands or feet, weakness.	You have had kidney problems.
May take several weeks before effective. Avoid alcohol. May impair ability to use heavy machinery. *Amitriptyline:* Do not take while taking MAO inhibitors. Inform dentists and surgeons when taking. May cause sun sensitivity. *Norpramin:* May cause anxiety, agitation, or other mental changes including suicidal thoughts.	Rapid heartbeat, constipation, dry mouth, blurred vision, drowsiness, dizziness, confusion, susceptibility to falls, nausea, sedation, vomiting, rash.	You have a history of heart or thyroid disease, urinary retention, glaucoma, seizure disorder. You develop confusion, blurred vision, heart palpitations, stiffness or trembling, problems urinating.
Potentially addictive; used only for short-term relief of moderate to severe pain. Avoid alcohol. Avoid tranquilizers and sedatives except under doctor's direction. Use caution while driving or operating heavy machinery. Potentially fatal drug reactions. *Demerol:* Do not take if you have been taking MAO inhibitors.	Dizziness, lightheadedness, nausea, sedation, sweating, vomiting. Less common: constipation, mood changes, rash. *Ultracet:* anorexia, prostate disorder.	You have a history of drug abuse or alcoholism, breathing disorders such as asthma or chronic obstructive pulmonary disease; head injury; liver, kidney, intestine, or prostate disorders; history of seizures. You develop slower breathing, faintness, confusion, any other unusual problems.

MAO = monoamine oxidase inhibitor.

* Dosages represent an average range for treatment of back pain. Precise dosage varies from person to person and depends on many factors. Do not make any change to your prescription medication without consulting your doctor.

† Available only as a generic.

Treating Back Pain

Fortunately, most episodes of back pain—about 90%—clear up with little or no treatment in about six weeks, reducing the need for medical intervention. As long as you are not experiencing severe back pain or other symptoms (such as severe nighttime pain or pain that worsens with lying down, weight loss, bowel or bladder dysfunction, or fever) that might indicate a health condition like cancer, infection, cauda equina syndrome, or an abdominal aortic aneurysm, you can safely try self-treatment.

Self-Treatment

You can take the following steps to help ease a backache.

Exercise

Back relaxation exercises—which involve gentle stretching to relax back muscles, lengthen the spine, and relieve compression of the vertebrae—are effective for alleviating stress and strain on the back. Ask your doctor for a referral to a physical therapist or for printed instructions on how to safely perform the exercises. Performing back exercises in water also can be beneficial (see "Working Out in Water" on pages 12-13).

Rest

Lying down takes pressure off the spine and usually lessens pain. The best postures in bed are lying in the fetal position with a pillow between the knees, or on your back with knees flexed, using a pillow to support the legs. Most experts advise limiting bed rest to one or two days, however. The inactivity associated with longer periods of bed rest may do more harm than good by weakening muscles.

It is better to get out of bed and move around as soon as you can do so with reasonable comfort, even if some pain persists. Until the pain fully disappears, you should avoid lifting, bending, vigorous exercise, or other activities that place stress on the back.

While it may seem risky to move around when you are still experiencing back pain, medical research supports limiting the amount of bed rest. One study, for instance, found that people with acute back pain who continued ordinary activities recovered more rapidly than those for whom bed rest was prescribed. In fact, within a week, just 20% of the normal-activity group were still absent from work, compared with 41% of those on bed rest. After three months, people in the bed-rest group accumulated an average of approximately nine sick days, compared with five sick days in the normal-activity group.

Ice

After a sudden back injury with pain limited to the back area, immediately applying ice can be therapeutic. In addition to relieving pain, ice reduces internal bleeding and swelling by decreasing blood flow.

An ice bag, commercial cold pack, or even a package of frozen vegetables should be used for 10 to 20 minutes every two hours for the first 48 hours after injury (while you're awake). The 20-minute limit is important to avoid the risk of frostbite. Another approach to relieving pain is to massage the painful area with an ice cube.

Heat

After an acute back injury, it is best to wait 48 hours before applying heat. But chronic back pain or a more widespread backache that begins some time after a back injury may be eased by relaxing muscles with a hot bath, a heating pad, a heat lamp, or hot, moist compresses.

Over-the-counter medications

Nonsteroidal anti-inflammatory drugs (NSAIDs)—such as aspirin, ibuprofen (Advil, Motrin), naproxen (Aleve), or ketoprofen (Orudis)—or the pain reliever acetaminophen (Tylenol) may help alleviate discomfort, reduce inflammation, or both. Be sure to read the labels and follow instructions carefully. Even over-the-counter medications can cause side effects if misused.

Traction, corsets, and braces

Little evidence supports the use of traction or corsets, although temporary use of a corset with built-in supports may be helpful during the recovery period following surgery or during activities that have to be performed even when you are still experiencing pain. Whether back braces help in treating back pain is unclear, and seemingly contradictory findings continue to be published.

Alternative Therapies

A major study on the use of alternative therapies found that almost 60% of people who consulted a medical doctor for back pain had tried some sort of alternative therapy. When contemplating one of these options, it is important to remember that the treatments are considered alternative precisely because there is not enough scientific evidence to prove that they work consistently. Be particularly cautious about undertaking any treatments that are expensive and require more than half a dozen visits.

Be sure to tell your doctor if you are using any type of alternative therapy. Commonly used alternative methods for relieving back pain include acupuncture, acupressure, massage, relaxation therapy, spinal manipulation, yoga, and biofeedback.

Acupuncture

This treatment is based on the traditional Chinese medical theory that pain and disease occur when the body's natural energies (chi) are out of balance. The Chinese believe that chi is conducted through the body along pathways called meridians, which intersect at specific points in the body. Stimulating these points through acupuncture needles is meant to correct the improper flow of chi, thereby relieving the problem.

Acupuncture is one of the few alternative therapies that are commonly covered by many insurance companies. Check with your insurer to be sure it covers this therapy.

The needles used in acupuncture are as thin as a hair. In general, 10 to 15 of these needles are inserted into the back to treat pain. Sometimes they are stimulated with electricity or heat or are turned after insertion. Acupuncture may relieve pain by triggering nerves to send out natural, pain-blocking chemicals (endorphins) within the body.

A recent analysis of 33 studies of acupuncture and back pain found that acupuncture effectively relieves chronic low back pain. But the researchers noted that there is no evidence that acupuncture is more effective than other therapies. To find a reputable practitioner, contact one of the acupuncture organizations listed on page 79.

Acupressure

This therapy is similar to acupuncture in that it is based on the same theory of energy channels in the body. Continuous pressure is exerted on a trigger spot for three to five minutes to stimulate the flow of healing energy. This pressure may temporarily alleviate the pain, but it usually returns.

Massage therapy

In addition to relaxing muscles and easing tension in the back, massage is believed to temporarily overpower pain signals going to the brain. Massage therapy should only be performed by a trained, licensed massage therapist.

Relaxation therapy

High levels of stress not only adversely affect overall health, but can also contribute to back pain. Relaxation therapy teaches muscle relaxation and breathing techniques for coping with the stress of everyday life.

Another relaxation technique is meditation, which is designed to calm the mind as well as the body. Researchers have theorized that the metabolic response to meditation—the opposite of the response to stress—may counter the negative effects of stress.

Biofeedback

Using electronic sensors, biofeedback measures a person's automatic, stress-responsive body functions—such as breathing patterns, pulse rate, and muscle tension—while the person practices different relaxation methods. Data from the sensors can show which relaxation techniques are most effective for that individual. Biofeedback can also help train a person to regulate his or her body functions consciously, reducing the impact of stress on the body.

Yoga

Mounting evidence suggests that yoga can relieve chronic back pain. There are many schools or types of yoga. They feature precise alignment and props such as mats, blocks, and straps. The props help in achieving correct yoga poses. The poses, combined with breathing techniques, help relax muscles and calm the mind.

Spinal manipulation

For treatment of back pain lasting less than a month, spinal manipulation can be a good choice, provided there is no evidence of a spinal nerve root disorder (such as a herniated disk or spinal stenosis) or fracture. If symptoms do not improve after four weeks, however, use of spinal manipulation should be re-evaluated.

A chiropractor, osteopath, or physical therapist may provide spinal manipulation, adjusting the vertebrae to reduce pain caused by poor alignment. The health care professional must be sure that back pain is not due to bone or joint disorders, since manipulating a spine that has been damaged by osteoporosis, for example, could result in further, more serious injury. X-rays of the area are usually taken before spinal manipulation to rule out vertebral fractures.

In properly screened people, spinal manipulation by a trained professional appears to be safe. Some people may experience discomfort, headache, or tiredness after treatment, but these effects are usually

When Back Pain Lingers

What you should know before you get an injection for persistent low back pain

Injection therapy is a fairly conservative alternative for the treatment of nagging low back pain. But the $64,000 question for doctors and patients alike is: Do injections really work? Before we answer that question, it's helpful to understand what's in the injections and where and when they may be used in people with persistent low back pain.

Injection Therapy: When, What, Where, and Why?
Injections may be given for low back pain that is subacute (lasting longer than one month) or chronic (lasting for three months or more). The shots typically contain a combination of an anesthetic (to numb pain) and a corticosteroid (to reduce inflammation).

The site of the injection in the spine varies depending on the suspected source of the pain. Your healthcare provider may use fluoroscopy (a type of x-ray movie in real time) or a CT scanner to help direct the needle to the correct location in the spinal column. Common injection sites are the:

Epidural space. An epidural injection with a corticosteroid is one of the most commonly used injection techniques. With this method, the steroid is injected directly into the epidural space (the area between the protective membrane of the spinal cord and the inner wall of the vertebrae).

Facet joint. Medication is injected into facet joints if they are suspected of being inflamed. These joints, located between vertebrae, enable the spine to bend and twist. Facet joint injections are also used as diagnostic tools to help identify the exact location of back pain.

Nerve root. Nerve roots emerge from the spinal column between vertebrae. Medication is injected over the area of the nerve thought to be inflamed.

Trigger point. Trigger points are locations where touch or pressure elicits pain at specific areas in a muscle. Medication is then injected into these tender spots.

So, Do They Work?
Maybe—at least in some people. Authors of a systematic review published last year in *Spine* took a look at 18 randomized, controlled trials—the gold standard of studies—of the effectiveness of injection therapy in nearly 1,200 people with subacute or chronic low back pain. Epidural, facet joint, and trigger point injections were reviewed. The studies analyzed excluded people who experienced leg pain and/or muscle weakness due to spinal nerve compression (radiculopathy).

More than one third (seven) of the 18 studies found that injection therapy was significantly more effective than placebo injections

only temporary. Serious complications of lower-spine manipulation, such as paralysis and death, are rare. Complications, when they do occur, are more common with manipulations of the neck.

Medical Treatment

If you have severe back pain that lasts more than a few days, or if you have mild to moderate back pain that does not respond to self-treatment, it is important to visit your primary care physician. Regardless of the cause of the pain, a doctor will probably recommend the self-treatment techniques described on pages 24-25. In general, limiting the amount of bed rest and pain medication is the preferred approach to back pain management among primary care physicians—a strategy supported by current research.

In one study of more than 1,000 people, doctors were divided into three groups according to whether they had a low, medium, or or other treatments, such as nonsteroidal anti-inflammatory drugs (NSAIDs), in providing short-term pain relief.

That means that in nearly two thirds of the studies, there was little evidence to suggest that injections were any more effective than placebo in providing short-term pain relief. In addition, none of the studies evaluated long-term effectiveness.

In spite of these findings, experts believe that it is still possible that certain subgroups of people with lingering low back pain could benefit from injection therapy. However, better-designed clinical trials are needed to determine just who those patients may be.

In the meantime, since injection therapy does appear to benefit some people, your doctor may suggest it as an option, particularly if other conservative therapies such as physical therapy have not been helpful and surgery is your next step.

Weighing the Risks and Benefits

Overall, injection therapy is a safe procedure, but adverse effects do sometimes occur. For example, nine of the 18 studies in the *Spine* review reported side effects, such as headache, dizziness, burning or tingling sensation, and nausea, in small numbers of people.

Some other adverse events to be aware of, although uncommon, include:

• bleeding or infection at the injection site

• spinal headache or postdural puncture headache—the needle puncture from an epidural injection may cause spinal fluid to leak from the epidural space. This changes the fluid pressure around the brain and spinal cord, which can cause a severe headache.

• neurological complications caused by damage to spinal nerves.

Keep in mind that serious complications from injection therapy for low back pain are rare, but they should always be taken into consideration.

Injection therapy is not suitable if you are susceptible to excessive bleeding or are taking anticoagulants (drugs that reduce the formation of blood clots). In addition, people experiencing pain due to infection or certain forms of cancer should not receive injections with steroids, since these drugs can weaken the immune system.

The Bottom Line

Most studies show that injection therapy is no more effective than placebo for subacute or chronic back pain. For some people, however, treatment can provide short-term pain relief. This temporary effect may be sufficient to enable you to take part in a physical therapy or exercise program, which can help alleviate the stress and strain on your back and get you back on your feet once again. ■

high frequency of prescribing pain medications and bed rest. After a month, people seeing the physicians who least often prescribed drugs and bed rest improved more quickly than those in the other groups. Only 30% of these people had to make moderate to severe cutbacks in their daily activities, compared with 37% of people seeing doctors in the medium-frequency group and 46% in the high-frequency group. After a year, however, there were no differences among the three groups in pain levels or ability to function.

Many doctors feel that the successful treatment of back pain with minimal bed rest and minimal medication is a result of the self-care practices they recommend. The above study supports this belief: People whose physicians were least likely to prescribe bed rest and pain-relief medications reported being more satisfied with their personal knowledge of how to treat back pain and just as satisfied with their medical care as those whose doctors prescribed drugs and rest.

Prescription NSAIDs

When over-the-counter medications do not relieve back pain, the doctor might need to prescribe a stronger NSAID such as diflunisal or meclofenamate (available in generic form only).

Although a certain type of NSAID known as COX-2 inhibitors have been shown to treat pain and inflammation as effectively as traditional NSAIDs, they have come under scrutiny for their adverse effects, including an increased risk of heart attack and stroke in individuals with or at risk for cardiovascular disease.

As a result of these concerns, the U.S. Food and Drug Administration (FDA) has strengthened the warnings on the labels of all NSAIDs, including the COX-2 inhibitor celecoxib (Celebrex). Currently, Celebrex is the only COX-2 inhibitor that remains on the market in the United States.

Muscle relaxants

Studies have shown that muscle relaxants are an effective treatment for low back pain of less than four weeks' duration. Their usefulness for chronic low back pain requires further study, however.

Muscle relaxants appear to work by depressing the activity of the nerves in the spinal cord and brain. Common muscle relaxants are baclofen (Lioresal), carisoprodol (Soma), cyclobenzaprine (Flexeril), and methocarbamol (Robaxin). The anticonvulsant gabapentin (Neurontin) also is used often. A few studies suggest that a combination of a muscle relaxant and an NSAID may be more beneficial than a muscle relaxant alone.

The use of muscle relaxants is controversial because they are potentially addictive. Therefore, you should not take them for more than one or two weeks, and people with a history of substance abuse or other mental health conditions should use them with great caution. Possible side effects include dizziness, drowsiness, dry mouth, headache, stomachache, and nausea or vomiting.

Epidural steroid injections

Epidural steroid injections may be used to treat low back pain and sciatica. The injections usually contain an anesthetic for pain relief and a corticosteroid, which helps to reduce inflammation around irritated nerves in the epidural space.

Studies have shown that epidural steroid injections can relieve back pain. Unfortunately, however, that relief is often only temporary. For more information about steroid injections for back pain, see "When Back Pain Lingers" on pages 28-29.

Opiates

Highly addictive painkillers such as opiates (morphine, codeine, meperidine) should also be used with a great deal of caution and only when all other treatments have failed. People who need opiates for more than a few days sometimes take controlled-release formulations of oxycodone (OxyContin) or morphine (MS Contin). These long-acting drugs provide more consistent control of back pain than standard, short-acting narcotics. (The chart on pages 22-23 gives an overview of oral medications prescribed for back pain.)

Disease-modifying antirheumatic drugs

The medication etanercept (Enbrel), a disease-modifying antirheumatic drug (DMARD), is used to treat ankylosing spondylitis. The drug works by interfering with an immune system protein known as tumor necrosis factor, which contributes to inflammation. Possible side effects of etanercept include reactions at the site of the injection, respiratory infections, and tuberculosis.

Exercise

If your back pain is mild, it is safe to get back to an aerobic exercise routine as soon as treatment eases your pain. After two weeks, exercises to strengthen the back and abdominal muscles can be started slowly. Building core strength in the back and abdomen is very beneficial in preventing recurrence.

Not recommended or unproven treatments

Prolonged bed rest (more than four days) is not recommended as part of treatment. Although still used occasionally, transcutaneous electrical nerve stimulation (TENS)—the application of low-energy electrical radiation to "numb" the nerves—is declining in popularity. Support belts and back machines have not been found to be of any benefit in the treatment of back pain.

Treating a Herniated Disk

Approximately 80 to 90% of people with classic symptoms of a herniated lumbar disk—sciatica and back spasm—respond within six weeks to rest and pain medication. This conservative approach to treatment likely works because it gives the swelling around the nerve root a chance to subside. The limitation on physical activity helps the herniated disk material remain in place, reducing the risk of it fragmenting. A disk fragment that lodges in the spinal canal and presses on a nerve can cause significant loss of function.

ASK THE DOCTOR

Q. ***I started having low back pain a couple of months ago, and I've had to be reassigned at my job. My doctor wants me to enroll in behavioral therapy sessions. Shouldn't I first see whether medication works?***

A. Although most people's low back pain resolves within four to six weeks, pain that doesn't respond within this period is more likely to become chronic. That's why it's important to seek effective treatment as soon as it becomes clear that the pain won't go away easily.

A 2009 study in the *Archives of Physical Medicine and Rehabilitation* looked at people with back pain that had begun six to 10 weeks earlier. A total of 67 people were randomized to receive either behavioral intervention, in which a clinician counseled participants on effective ways to cope with pain, or a control group in which clinicians provided support but no specific suggestions. All participants also received standard care, such as medication and physical therapy.

They study found that people assigned to behavioral intervention were more likely than those in the control group to be recovered after six months (52% versus 31%).

If your doctor is recommending behavioral therapy, it's important to give it a try. It could very well make the difference between recovery and living with chronic back pain.

Surgery

Surgery for a herniated disk may be unavoidable in people who experience impaired bowel or bladder function, persistent or increasing sciatica despite bed rest, progressive leg weakness, and recurring episodes of incapacitating pain from sciatica.

Diskectomy. The traditional surgical treatment of a herniated disk, called diskectomy, is used only when at least six weeks of nonsurgical treatment offers no pain relief or when there is a problem in nerve function that causes a loss of movement, known as a neurological deficit. The procedure relieves pressure on the pinched nerve by making an incision into the distended annulus fibrosus (the tough outer layers of the disk) and removing the protruding nucleus pulposus (the gel-like center). General anesthesia is required. Depending on the location of the herniation, the surgeon may need to remove a small part of the vertebra (open laminectomy) to gain access to the herniation site.

In general, diskectomy produces improvement more rapidly than conservative treatment. The long-term results of surgical and nonsurgical treatment, however, are about the same. How well you do during the first three months of conservative care may help you decide about surgery. If your pain is tolerable, you may be able to get by without it. But if the pain is intolerable, then surgery becomes a more attractive option because it can dramatically reduce the pain.

One day of hospitalization may be required after having an open diskectomy (a procedure in which the surgeon makes a large incision in the patient's back to gain access to and operate on the spine). Over the subsequent several weeks, the treated disk gradually restabilizes as scar tissue fills the empty space. Almost all people can return to work six to eight weeks after the operation. Repeat surgery is not as effective at relieving pain as the first surgery (see "What's Next When Back Surgery Fails?" on pages 34-35).

Spinal fusion. In some cases, a spinal fusion is also performed. This procedure involves using bone grafts to fuse together two or more adjacent vertebrae. It should be considered when chronic back pain was present before the herniated disk led to leg pain. Spinal fusion is not always reliable, and guidelines as to when it should be done are not as clear as those for diskectomy. Fusion may be recommended when back pain is greater than leg pain and is chronic. It is also recommended when a repeat operation is necessary because the first one was not effective in relieving pain or because herniation has recurred. Unfortunately, spinal fusion alters the way the spine moves and may promote degenerative changes as well.

Artificial disks. Although artificial disks have been available in Europe for at least 20 years, the FDA did not approve their use in the United States until 2004. The first artificial disk available in this country, called the Charité, was authorized for use in single-level disk problems (where one disk is affected) after clinical trials revealed that the device preserved motion and was as effective as spinal fusion in relieving pain, with shorter healing and rehabilitation times. In 2006, the FDA approved a second artificial spinal disk, the ProDisc-L.

Additional artificial disks are being tested in clinical trials in the United States. However, it will take five to 10 years to determine whether artificial disks can maintain long-term motion and prevent disk degeneration near the surgical site.

Candidates for disk surgery should have degeneration in only one disk in the lumbar spine with little or no arthritis in the corresponding facet joints; have undergone at least six months of conservative treatment, such as use of pain medication or physical therapy, with no improvement in symptoms; not have significant leg pain; and be in overall good health.

Minimally invasive procedures. There are several less-invasive surgical alternatives that allow a smaller incision than traditional surgery.

• ***Microdiskectomy*** is performed by the surgeon using very small precision instruments placed inside an endoscope (a small lighted tube) and inserted through a miniscule opening in the back. The surgeon can view the disk and nerves through the endoscope as well as remove herniated disk material.

Microdiskectomy appears to have a success rate similar to that of open diskectomy. Doctors may recommend this surgery to people who have leg pain for at least six weeks but do not experience relief with conservative treatments such as oral corticosteroids, NSAIDs, and physical therapy.

• ***Percutaneous arthroscopic diskectomy*** involves inserting a probe into the spine to scoop out the disk.

• ***Intradiskal electrothermal therapy*** (IDET) involves inserting a wire into the back that transmits heat into the collagen fibers of the disk, destroying pain receptors in the area. IDET initially appeared promising, but more recent reports have been disappointing.

• ***Laser diskectomy*** uses a laser to burn out the disk. This procedure has been the subject of considerable debate, as the results of the procedure have varied greatly. Some studies show no greater improvement in symptoms after laser diskectomy than in similar cases where no surgery was performed; in others, it is as successful as standard surgery.

ASK THE DOCTOR

Q. ***I'm considering having an artificial disk implanted for lower back pain. Is this a better option than spinal fusion?***

A. Early studies have shown that artificial disks work as well as spinal fusion, and they can be a good option for people whose pain originates solely from an intervertebral disk. The devices were developed in an attempt to avoid the stiffness that spinal fusion causes, potentially leading to increased stress and degeneration in the adjacent areas of the spine.

The devices have not been proven to work better than spinal fusion, although one recent study from Sweden suggested that they might. The study, published in the *European Spine Journal* in 2009, randomly assigned 152 men and women to either disk replacement or spinal fusion. After two years, people who had received an artificial disk were twice as likely as those who had undergone spinal fusion to be completely free of pain (30% versus 15%). The majority of people in this study (67%) were either "much better" or completely free of pain after two years, meaning that results with either procedure were quite good.

Doctors still don't know how well artificial disks will hold up after five or 10 years. What's more, artificial disks are expensive and generally not covered by insurance. Ask your doctor which procedure is best for you.

What's Next When Back Surgery Fails?

Managing disabling back pain after unsuccessful surgery

For some people, surgery noticeably improves or eliminates back pain once and for all. Unfortunately, however, a good number of patients do not experience such a successful outcome. In fact, up to 40% continue to suffer from chronic back pain after undergoing spinal surgery. Doctors and researchers describe such cases as "failed back surgery syndrome."

What should you do if back surgery fails to eliminate your pain? Unfortunately, there is no single or simple answer. One person's situation and treatment can differ vastly from the next's. More often than not, however, finding pain relief will require input from a multidisciplinary team of healthcare providers that may include your primary care physician, a surgeon, a physical therapist, and, perhaps, a mental health professional and a pain management specialist.

What's Causing the Pain?

One of the first things your doctor will do is try to find the cause of the recurring pain. Interestingly, it may not be the same as the problem for which you initially had surgery. How soon the pain recurs after surgery and the type of surgical procedure you had can provide valuable information about the potential cause. Your doctor may also order imaging studies such as magnetic resonance imaging (MRI) and computed tomography (CT).

Early onset. If pain continues following back surgery or recurs very soon after, it could be due to the surgical procedure itself. One possibility is that the site operated on was not the sole cause of the pain. For example, pain may persist because the surgery addressed a problem in a particular vertebra but not in the adjacent disk. Alternatively, a herniated disk or spinal stenosis that was seen on an MRI or CT scan and operated on by the surgeon was not responsible for your back pain after all.

If you had a laminectomy, continuing pain may be a sign that the spinal canal was not sufficiently enlarged during decompression surgery to completely relieve pressure on the nerve. Another possibility: A disk fragment was not adequately removed and is still pinching a nerve.

Pain subsiding initially but then recurring within a few weeks of surgery could also be a sign of infection.

Intermediate onset. Back pain that returns several months after surgery may indicate a reherniated disk, an inflamed nerve root, or formation of scar tissue near the nerve root. Arachnoiditis also may be suspected. This is a disorder that arises from inflammation of the membrane that surrounds and protects the spinal nerves, leading to clumping of the nerves and chronic pain.

Late onset. Pain that occurs several years after surgery may be due to the recurrence of spinal stenosis. It might also indicate the loss of spinal stability at or adjacent to the surgical site. This problem can develop when too much bone is removed during decompression surgery or after spinal fusion surgery when adjacent vertebrae overcompensate for the loss of motion at the fused vertebrae.

Repeat Back Surgery

Your doctor may recommend another operation if an infection develops, you lose control of your bladder or bowel function, you experience nerve damage that gets progressively worse, the hardware used during fusion surgery breaks, loosens, or irritates nerves, or nonunion develops.

In general, however, nonsurgical options will be tried first, as the chances of a successful outcome often decrease with each subsequent surgery. If nonsurgical measures aren't helpful and the pain is keeping you from performing normal daily activities, surgery will be considered—but only if your imaging study shows a specific structural defect, such as spinal stenosis or disk herniation, is causing the problem. If no specific cause of pain is seen on CT or MRI, surgery will not be performed.

Nonsurgical Options

Several nonsurgical treatment options may be tried after failed back surgery. Oral pain medication and physical therapy are typically the first steps.

Oral pain medication. First-line therapy for failed back surgery syndrome is usually daily use of a prescription-strength nonsteroidal anti-inflammatory drug (NSAID) such as naproxen (Naprosyn) or celecoxib (Celebrex).

To protect against the development of ulcers and internal bleeding, which can occur with regular NSAID use, your doctor may also prescribe a proton pump inhibitor, such as esomeprazole (Nexium), omeprazole (Prilosec), or lansoprazole (Prevacid). Because NSAIDs can also raise the likelihood of heart attack and stroke in people who have or are at risk for cardiovascular disease, you and your doctor should carefully weigh the benefits of these drugs against their risks.

Your doctor may also prescribe a tricyclic antidepressant like amitriptyline or desipramine (Norpramin). Not only are antidepressants in this class effective for treating depression, they also help reduce the sensation of pain.

Another option is a narcotic pain reliever such as hydrocodone, oxycodone, or morphine. Because narcotic drugs are addictive, they are typically used only for short-term relief of severe pain.

In rare cases, intraspinal drug delivery may help. With this system, a miniature pump implanted beneath the skin of the abdomen continuously infuses small amounts of pain medication directly into the cerebrospinal fluid. In this way, a much lower dose is delivered to the brain, which reduces side effects while providing pain relief.

Physical therapy. This treatment option is important to reduce pain and improve function. Physical therapy typically involves exercises to strengthen the muscles of the abdomen and back and is often part of a rehabilitation program that also includes occupational therapy and psychological counseling. Studies show that these comprehensive programs are more effective than physical therapy alone.

Epidural steroid injections. These injections have been used for many years for nerve-related back pain. While some studies show them to provide effective pain relief for people with failed back surgery syndrome, others do not. To date, no randomized, controlled trials—the gold standard of studies—have compared epidural steroid injections with a repeat operation.

Spinal cord stimulation. With spinal cord stimulation, tiny electrodes implanted along the spinal cord deliver a small electrical current that interrupts the nerve impulses that carry pain signals to the brain. Several studies—although few randomized, controlled trials—have been conducted, and they show that spinal cord stimulation is effective in people with failed back surgery syndrome.

A recent review of several studies showed that stimulators reduced pain by at least 50% in about one third of patients. By comparison, similar levels of pain reduction were achieved by only 10% of those who had a repeat operation. However, one randomized, controlled trial reported that 34% of people who received the implants experienced problems such as infections or equipment malfunctions.

In addition, spinal cord stimulation will not permanently eliminate the pain, but an evaluation of studies by the American Society of Interventional Pain Physicians found strong evidence that it provides short-term (less than one year) relief and moderate evidence that it offers longer-term relief.

Radiofrequency neurolysis. This procedure temporarily destroys targeted spinal nerves using heat. The heat is applied via an electrode that is guided through an insulated needle. This procedure can reduce pain for as long as three years. However, there are no studies comparing it to reoperation.

Coping Strategies Can Help

If you have back pain after surgery—even when a specific source cannot be identified—it doesn't mean the pain is not real or is "all in your head." Still, it's common for persistent pain and an inability to perform daily activities to adversely affect your emotional state. Many people with chronic, disabling pain experience depression, anxiety, and sleep disturbances, which, in turn, can amplify the perception of pain.

Studies show that psychological counseling helps. In sessions, you'll learn how to manage the way you respond to chronic pain and identify thoughts and behaviors that may worsen it. For this type of help, you can see a mental health professional with experience in chronic pain, or you may prefer a multidisciplinary program that offers counseling as part of its rehabilitative services. (See Pain Treatment Facilities, on pages 40-41).

The Road Ahead

The road to pain relief may be bumpy following failed back surgery. To find the right treatment, you'll need to have frank discussions with your doctor. Ask lots of questions to make sure you understand the full range of feasible treatment options, along with their risks and benefits. It's also crucial to have realistic expectations regarding potential outcomes, so ask what level of function and pain you can expect after surgery. Only with this information in hand can you make an informed choice about your next steps. ■

Treating Vertebral Compression Fractures

The treatment of vertebral compression fractures includes minimal bed rest, pain medication, exercise, and osteoporosis treatment to reduce the risk of future fractures. In some cases, surgical procedures such as percutaneous vertebroplasty, kyphoplasty, or spinal fusion are performed.

Treating Spinal Stenosis

Nonsurgical treatment is appropriate if the symptoms of spinal stenosis are mild or if a person is not a good candidate for surgery—for example, an older adult who also has another serious illness. Treatment includes pain relievers such as acetaminophen (Tylenol) or NSAIDs, weight loss, and, especially, exercises to increase flexibility. Some success has been reported with the use of caudal epidural blocks—injections of pain relievers and a steroid directly into the base of the spine. If these measures fail to control symptoms, surgery is considered. Surgery is necessary when severe neurological deficits or impaired bowel or bladder function develop.

Surgical treatment

Decompression surgery for spinal stenosis enlarges the spinal canal to relieve pressure on the spinal cord. After the spinal column is opened at the narrowed points, the bone or fibrous tissue responsible for the constriction is removed. At times, a disk or fragments of a disk also may be removed. If an extensive amount of bone is removed, it may be necessary to fuse together two or more vertebrae to stabilize the spinal column (this may slightly decrease a person's flexibility).

The hospital stay for decompression surgery is typically three to five days. A person can get around using a walker the first or second day and then graduate to a cane, which he or she uses for six to 12 weeks. After that, walking without assistance is usually possible. Results tend to be excellent if the disease is limited to one or two vertebrae. Studies have shown that leg pain associated with stenosis significantly improves after surgery in 70 to 85% of people. For information on options when surgery is not successful, see "What's Next When Back Surgery Fails?" on pages 34-35.

Risks of surgery

Older adults with spinal stenosis may have other health conditions, such as heart disease or arthritis, that increase the risk of surgical complications. These conditions do not necessarily rule out surgery as a treatment option, however.

In one study, investigators monitored 50 people, age 71 to 84, who had undergone decompression surgery. Half of the people had other disorders that severely limited their mobility. No complications involving anesthesia, the heart, or blood clots occurred during the procedure. After two years, 28 of the study participants (more than half) rated the procedure's effect on their leg pain as excellent (almost or totally pain free); nine reported fair relief (improved but residual pain); and nine said their pain was unchanged. Although the operation provided some relief, the rates of excellent outcomes were not as high as researchers had hoped. Therefore, although having other health conditions did not cause additional complications, it appeared to reduce the chances of obtaining the best results.

Treating Paget's Disease

Many people with Paget's disease require no treatment because they have no symptoms. The most clear-cut reasons for using drugs to treat Paget's disease are bone pain, bone fractures (such as vertebral fractures), and compression of nerves in the spine or elsewhere.

The FDA has approved injectable calcitonin, four oral bisphosphonate drugs (a class of drugs used to strengthen bone), and two intravenous bisphosphonate drugs for treatment of Paget's disease. Calcitonin (a synthetic version of a hormone that acts on bone) has pain-relieving properties and may be used in conjunction with a bisphosphonate, especially if additional pain relief is desired. No matter which drug is started first, it can be discontinued and replaced with another agent if it proves ineffective.

Calcitonin

Calcitonin (Miacalcin), which inhibits bone breakdown (resorption), is available for subcutaneous (under the skin) or intramuscular injection. Although it is also available as a nasal spray, the nasal formulation of calcitonin is not approved by the FDA for treating Paget's disease. Injections are initially given daily; after a month or so, symptoms may be controlled with less frequent injections (three times a week, for example).

After a variable period of time, calcitonin stops working in some people. Between 10 and 20% of those treated with calcitonin develop nausea, loss of appetite, and flushing of the face and ears.

Bisphosphonates

The bisphosphonate class of drugs includes the oral medications alendronate (Fosamax), etidronate (Didronel), risedronate (Actonel),

NEW RESEARCH

Vertebroplasty Appears To Be Ineffective in Short Term

Vertebroplasty, in which a surgeon injects medical-grade cement into the spine, is a recommended treatment for fractures that don't respond to medication. But a new study finds that vertebroplasty doesn't work any better than a sham procedure, at least in the short term.

The study included 131 people with one to three painful vertebral compression fractures caused by osteoporosis. Participants were randomly assigned to have either vertebroplasty or a sham procedure in which no cement was injected.

Participants in both groups reported improvements in pain and disability immediately after the procedure. A month later, the improvements in pain and disability remained similar in both groups. There was some indication that people in the vertebroplasty group had greater improvements in pain, but the small size of the study made it impossible to know whether the difference was real or simply occurred by chance.

If you're considering vertebroplasty, you should be aware that the benefits of this procedure are in doubt. What's more, cement leakage can cause problems like soft-tissue damage and nerve-root pain. Always discuss the potential benefits and risks of any procedure in detail with your doctor.

THE NEW ENGLAND JOURNAL OF MEDICINE
Volume 361, page 569
August 6, 2009

and tiludronate (Skelid). These drugs are the first line of therapy for the treatment of Paget's disease, and they are also used to prevent and treat osteoporosis.

For Paget's disease, alendronate (40 mg a day) and etidronate (200-400 mg a day) are both taken in a six-months-on, six-months-off cycle. Risedronate (30 mg a day) is taken in a two-months-on, two-months-off cycle and tiludronate (400 mg a day) is taken in a three-months-on, three-months-off cycle. If relapse occurs, a person may begin treatment again after two or three months off the drug.

If an oral bisphosphonate is no longer effective or cannot be tolerated because of gastrointestinal side effects or if Paget's disease is particularly severe, the intravenous bisphosphonate drugs pamidronate (Aredia) and zoledronic acid (Reclast) may be used. Reclast was approved by the U.S. Food and Drug Administration in April 2007 for the treatment of Paget's disease. Previously, zoledronic acid had been approved under the brand name Zometa for the treatment of cancer-related bone problems.

Pamidronate is administered using an injection schedule determined by the doctor. Possible side effects include abdominal cramps, chills, fever, nausea, pain, muscle spasms, sore throat, and muscle stiffness. Zoledronic acid is given in one 15-minute intravenous infusion. Potential side effects are similar to those of pamidronate.

Additional treatments

People with Paget's disease should also take 1,000 to 1,200 mg of calcium and 400 IU of vitamin D each day. People with signs and symptoms of spinal stenosis resulting from Paget's disease may require surgery if medication is ineffective in reducing the stenosis.

Treating Spinal Deformities

Most spinal deformities in adults, including adults over age 50, can be helped with flexibility exercises, posture maintenance, and general fitness. Mild anti-inflammatory medication and, occasionally, a rigid brace may help, although many older people cannot tolerate braces.

Surgery is recommended if the deformity is severe or will continue to worsen with age, if there are neurological problems associated with the deformity, or if pain does not respond to other measures.

Surgery usually involves the application of internal implants fixed to the bone (which allow for partial correction of the deformity) together with a spinal fusion. Old age should not prevent you from having this surgery if you need it, provided you are in good general health. Results are satisfactory 85% of the time.

Treating Cancer

Although myeloma and metastatic cancer cannot be cured, palliative treatment of back pain is often possible. Palliative care refers to treatment aimed at relieving pain and limiting any complications of a disease, rather than treatment aimed at curing a disease. Palliative treatment of back pain may include chemotherapy, radiation directed at the site of tumor invasion, and, at times, surgery.

For metastatic cancer of the spine, surgery may provide significant pain relief and preserve or restore nerve function. Bisphosphonate drugs are also used to reduce pain in metastatic cancer. People with metastatic prostate cancer may benefit from hormone therapies.

Managing Chronic Back Pain

Most back pain resolves in a few weeks to months; however, for some individuals the pain becomes a constant that interferes with daily life. If ignored, chronic back pain—unremitting pain that lasts at least six months and is not relieved by standard treatments—can lead to depression, disturbed sleep, poor balance, withdrawal from physical and social activities, inability to work, and reduced quality of life.

The first step in relieving chronic back pain is careful medical evaluation by a doctor to assess the nature and degree of the pain and, if possible, to pinpoint the cause. Because pain is a subjective experience, the doctor will ask when and how often the pain occurs; what brings it on and how long it lasts; its location, intensity, and quality (for example, is it sharp, dull, or tingling?); and what treatments you have tried and how well they have worked. You may also be asked to rate the severity of your pain on a standard pain scale.

If your doctor is not able to identify a specific cause for the pain (such as nerve entrapment that can be relieved by surgery), a variety of medications may be tried, ranging from over-the-counter acetaminophen or NSAIDs to prescription antidepressants, muscle relaxants, or opiates (see the chart on pages 22-23).

Weight loss (if necessary) and exercise—stretching, flexibility, and muscle-strengthening exercises—are helpful in treating chronic pain. Other strategies that may be useful include self-application of heat and cold and cognitive and/or behavioral therapy. Spinal manipulation, acupuncture, acupressure, massage, relaxation therapy, or biofeedback may also help. If these measures fail to relieve the pain, your doctor may advise you to enroll in a pain treatment facility.

NEW RESEARCH

Benefits of Spondylolisthesis Surgery Persist Over Time

Surgery is known to have short-term benefits over nonsurgical treatment for spondylolisthesis. Now, a study finds that benefits persist even after four years.

In a two-part study called the Spine Patient Research Trial (SPORT), researchers studied more than 600 people with spondylolisthesis. For the first part, researchers randomized 304 people to either surgery or nonoperative care. A total of 66% of the surgery group and 54% of the nonoperative group had surgery by the four-year point. For the second part, researchers observed 303 participants. Of these, 97% of people who chose surgery received it and 33% of those who chose nonoperative care also underwent surgery.

The differences between groups in the randomized study were not significantly different after four years, which is unsurprising given that so many people in the nonoperative group wound up having surgery. But when the researchers looked specifically at those who had actually undergone surgery, they saw significantly better scores for pain, physical function, overall patient satisfaction, and self-rated progress compared with those who received nonoperative treatment.

Although surgery always has risks, this study suggests that it may provide lasting benefits for people with spondylolisthesis.

THE JOURNAL OF BONE AND JOINT SURGERY (AMERICAN VOLUME)
Volume 91-A, page 1295
June 2009

Pain Treatment Facilities

Thousands of pain treatment facilities in the United States offer programs for individuals with chronic pain, including back pain. These programs do not aim to cure the cause of pain. Rather, they take advantage of a variety of approaches to reduce or eliminate pain and its negative effects on daily life.

People generally turn to pain treatment facilities when they have run out of other options. These facilities can help individuals living with chronic pain to improve both their physical and mental coping skills. The programs focus on managing the following:

- Pain behavior—actions that worsen the quality of life, such as limping, moaning, moving slowly, or using a cane
- Self perception—perceiving oneself as impaired or having a disability
- Pain perception—a discrepancy between how much pain a person feels and how much his or her condition typically produces
- Mental health problems—depression, anxiety, drug or alcohol dependence (about 25% of chronic pain sufferers become dependent on pain-control medication), and impaired memory or concentration.

Pain facilities are generally not advised for individuals who have unstable medical conditions (for example, uncontrolled high blood pressure or heart failure) or unrealistic expectations (such as finding a total cure) or for those who are unwilling to participate in a formal program.

There are several types of pain facilities. Some focus on a single treatment method, such as acupuncture, while others target pain in a particular region of the body. There are also multidisciplinary pain centers or clinics, which doctors usually prefer because they offer a more comprehensive approach and have shown superior results in medical studies. Multidisciplinary centers view pain as a complex syndrome. Therefore, they provide an integrated treatment team that generally includes a primary care physician, surgeon, psychologist or psychiatrist, nurse, physical therapist, occupational therapist, vocational counselor, and social worker.

Since the quality of care varies from one program to another, finding the right one can take some time. Your physician may be able to recommend a facility, or you can contact the Commission on Accreditation of Rehabilitation Facilities, which will provide a list of accredited programs in your area (see page 79 for contact information). Although accreditation is not required, accredited programs tend to be comprehensive. In addition, some insurance plans cover only accredited facilities. The American Pain Society also can provide information about pain centers in your vicinity (see page 79). In addition, the following tips may be helpful in your search:

• Programs located in hospitals and rehabilitation centers are most likely to offer comprehensive treatment. For the most specialized care, they should be located in a separate unit specifically set aside for the pain program.

• A good chronic pain program should include most of these features: biofeedback training, individual and family counseling, group therapy, occupational therapy, assertiveness training, regional anesthesia (nerve blocks), physical therapy, relaxation training and stress management, educational programs on medication and other aspects of pain management, and follow-up care after program completion.

• Make sure the program encourages family involvement. Educational sessions and joint counseling for your family members can help them to better understand your pain and the best ways to support you.

• Find out what services your health insurance policy will reimburse.

• Try to meet with several staff members before you enter a program. The medical director should have board certification and training in pain management. Ask about the physical setup, whether the program is inpatient or outpatient, the duration of the program (and length of any inpatient stay), and whether job retraining is involved. You may also consider asking whether any current participants would be willing to speak to you about their experience.

• Make sure the program reviews your previous medical records and gives you a complete physical exam before entry. Bring copies of your recent medical records.

Neck Pain

The cervical spine, located in the neck, is subject to many of the same problems that plague the lower back—muscle strains and spasms, disk degeneration and denervation, and spinal stenosis. About 10 to 15% of people experience neck pain at any given time. Most neck pain is short lived and gets better on its own or with simple self-care measures. But sometimes neck pain is a red flag for a more serious problem.

NEW RESEARCH

Traditional Rehabilitation Very Effective for Back Pain

Traditional rehabilitation is "very effective" for chronic back pain, according to a new study. Adding a behavioral component to treatment has only a small effect.

In the study, 363 patients with chronic back pain were randomly assigned to one of three groups. People in the traditional therapy group received three weeks of standard orthopedic rehabilitation. Those in the combined group received standard rehabilitation plus four weeks of psychological support and strategies for coping with pain. Those in the extended group received the same treatment as those in the combined group, with continued psychological support for up to a year.

All three treatments were effective at improving scores on various measures of pain. People in the combined and extended groups improved slightly more than those in the traditional rehabilitation group, but only on measures of depression and several coping strategies. Results were not significantly better in the extended group than in the combined group.

Chronic pain has a psychological component, which is why researchers thought that behavioral treatment might have a major effect on chronic back pain. Although this study doesn't support the need for routine behavioral treatment, it's possible that certain subgroups of people might benefit from it.

CLINICAL JOURNAL OF PAIN
Volume 25, page 356
June 2009

Causes

The neck supports the weight of the head, which can weigh 10 lbs or more. Although the head should be centered over the spine when we sit or stand upright, countless activities—such as sitting at a computer, reading, watching television, or eating—cause people to slump, rounding their upper back and tilting their head forward. This posture can lead to muscle strain or spasm in the neck. Muscle strain or spasm can also arise from constantly looking over or under one's glasses, having poor sleeping posture, or taking extended car trips.

General wear and tear from everyday activities and normal aging can cause changes in the disks of the neck that lead to pain and stiffness. For example, herniation of the intervertebral disks in the neck can decrease the space through which nerves exit the spinal canal, leading to pinched nerves and consequent pain. Bony outgrowths on the vertebrae (called osteophytes) also can pinch nerves. Spinal stenosis can put pressure on the spinal cord, causing pain or paralysis. Most people with neck pain do not have a herniated disk, osteophytes, or a disease that affects the spinal cord. Typically, it is the result of muscle strain or spasm, as described on page 4.

On occasion, neck pain can result from acceleration/deceleration injuries, commonly known as whiplash. It can also stem from serious problems like arthritis or cancer or from problems that originate in other areas of the body such as the shoulder. Chronic neck pain that is not associated with any physical problem may result from associated stress or depression.

When To See a Doctor

Many cases of neck pain get better on their own. If neck pain is linked to a recent recreational or work-related activity, the pain will likely decrease within two weeks, and treatment from a doctor is usually unnecessary. However, you should see a doctor if your neck pain follows a serious injury or is accompanied by the following:

- headaches, fever, or weight loss
- pain that worsens at night
- difficulty walking, clumsiness, or weakness
- pain, numbness, or tingling in your fingers, arms, or legs
- problems with bladder, bowel, or sexual function
- discomfort or pressure in your chest
- severe pain over a bone that might indicate a fracture or injury to a ligament
- osteoporosis or extended corticosteroid treatment (increases your risk of fracture).

Also see your doctor if your pain lasts longer than two weeks. Waiting too long before seeing the doctor for neck pain decreases the likelihood that the pain will completely resolve.

Diagnosis

If you do seek help for neck pain from a physician, your evaluation will include a medical history, a physical examination, and, if needed, imaging tests. During the physical exam, the doctor will likely measure your reflexes, range of motion, sensation, strength, and muscle and nerve function in your neck, arms, and legs.

If pain is the only symptom, and it does not radiate beyond your neck, imaging studies are usually not necessary. In this case, the pain is likely temporary and requires no invasive treatment. However, for people with a traumatic injury, rheumatoid arthritis, or a physical exam that does not pin down the cause of the pain, imaging studies may be needed. Imaging tests include x-rays, MRI scans, and CT scans. Further options may include electromyography and nerve conduction tests to assess the combined function of the muscles and nerves. People with intense pain that lasts for months may need further evaluation to rule out cancer.

Treatment

Early treatment of neck pain is recommended to prevent long-term disability. For neck pain that is not severe, noninvasive measures are generally tried first, beginning with over-the-counter medications such as acetaminophen (Tylenol) to treat pain or NSAIDs for pain and inflammation. Applying cold (especially in the initial stages of pain) and heat (in the later stages) can be helpful. Bed rest, reducing physical activity, and immobilizing the neck with a cervical collar may relieve pain in some people. (Cervical collars are available at surgical supply stores but should be used for no more than 10 days to avoid weakening the neck muscles.)

Range-of-motion exercises and massage also can be helpful. A physical therapist can teach you appropriate neck stretches and exercises for the shoulders and upper back to help ease neck pain and prevent future episodes. Your doctor or physical therapist may also instruct you on how to correct detrimental aspects of your posture or the setup of your office.

If two weeks of conservative treatment do not alleviate the pain, muscle relaxants, ongoing physical therapy, or spinal manipulation (chiropractic) may be recommended. Another treatment option is a cervical traction device, which uses a system of weights and pulleys to

NEW RESEARCH

Exercise Therapy Underutilized For Chronic Back and Neck Pain

Current guidelines recommend the use of exercise therapy for treating chronic back and neck pain. Yet according to a new study, exercise is not being prescribed enough in everyday practice.

The study involved administering a telephone survey to 684 individuals who had visited a healthcare professional for chronic back or neck pain in the previous 12 months. Only about half of the people had received a prescription for exercise therapy.

People were more likely to receive a prescription for exercise if they had seen a physical therapist or chiropractor than if they had seen a physician or other healthcare professional. Another difference was that physical therapists provided more supervision and prescribed more strengthening exercises than physicians and chiropractors. They also prescribed more stretching exercises than physicians.

Research indicates that people with chronic low back or neck pain exercise therapy benefit most from an exercise program with supervision. No matter who you see about your painful neck and back, be sure to ask whether you could benefit from a supervised exercise program.

ARTHRITIS & RHEUMATISM (ARTHRITIS CARE & RESEARCH)
Volume 61, page 192
February 15, 2009

help relieve pressure on the neck. The device is available at surgical supply stores.

For individuals whose neck pain appears to be caused by stress or depression, stress-management techniques, antidepressants, or both are often useful. In addition, your doctor may prescribe corticosteroid medications (either oral or injected) to reduce inflammation.

Even people with disk herniation or mild spinal stenosis should be treated first with conservative measures if the pain does not radiate beyond the neck. If no treatment has relieved the neck pain after eight weeks or if imaging studies indicate serious structural problems, you may need to consult with a spinal surgeon (a neurosurgeon or an orthopedic surgeon). Surgery involves relieving pressure on the spinal cord or the pinched nerve. Up to 90% of people who undergo surgery for neck pain experience significant pain relief.

OSTEOPOROSIS

The word osteoporosis means porous bone. A person with osteoporosis typically has low bone mass, poor bone quality, and fragile bones. This combination, together with the increased risk of falling among older people, leads to painful fractures and other health problems.

About 10 million Americans—eight million women and two million men—already have osteoporosis, and 34 million more are at increased risk because of low bone mass (osteopenia). Osteoporosis-related fractures are estimated to account for $19 billion in hospital and nursing home costs each year, and these costs are increasing. As our population continues to age (more than 35% of Americans will be age 50 or older by 2011), osteoporosis is expected to become an even greater health problem.

Structure of the Bones

Bones are not static, solid structures that do not change over time, although that's what many people think. Bone is actually a living tissue that undergoes a constant process of renewal and rebuilding. In this process, called bone remodeling, old bone is resorbed (broken down) and new bone is formed (see the illustration on page 45).

The framework of each bone is a matrix (scaffold) that is primarily composed of collagen. Collagen is soft but hardens as calcium and phosphorus are deposited. A regular supply of these minerals, which

How Bones Form and Repair

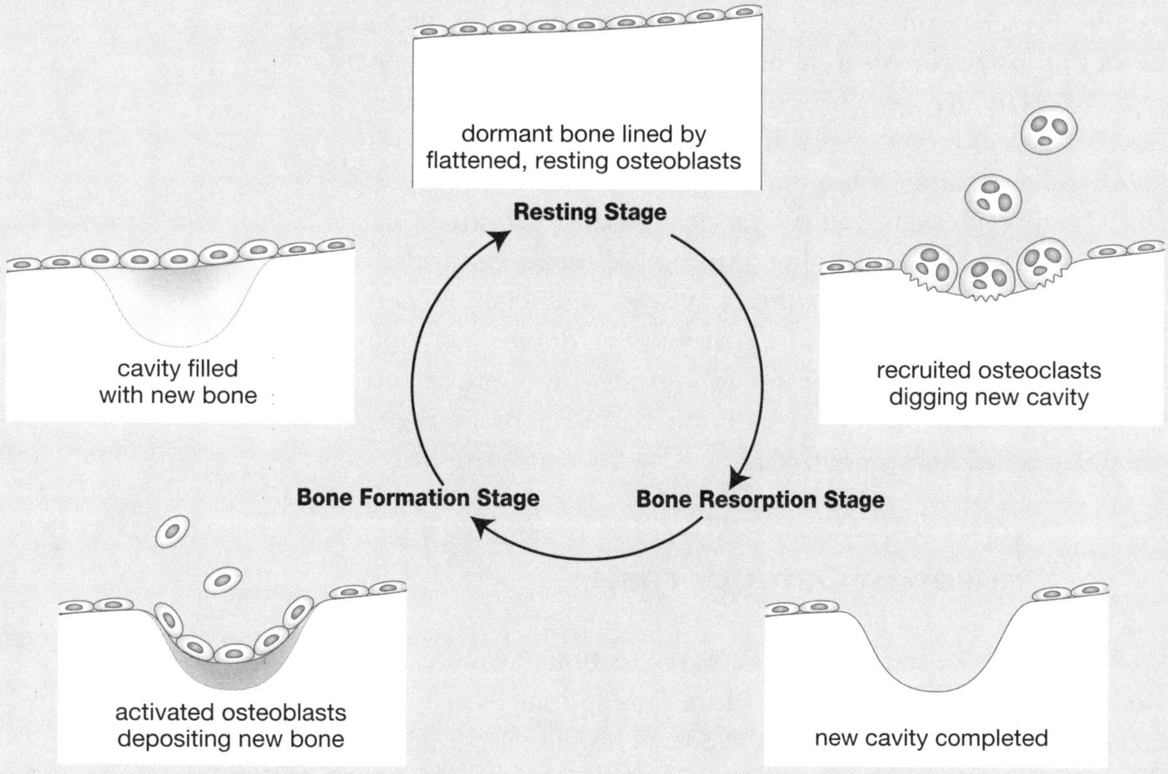

Many people think of their bones as stable structures that do not change with time. But bone is a living tissue that undergoes a constant process of renewal. In this process, called bone remodeling, old bone is resorbed (broken down) and new bone is formed.

The framework of each bone is a matrix, or scaffold, that is mostly made up of collagen. Although collagen is soft, it hardens with the deposition of calcium and phosphorus, which enter the bone from the bloodstream. A regular supply of these minerals is required to keep bones strong.

In the resorption stage of bone remodeling, special cells called osteoclasts invade the surface of the bone and remove both the matrix and minerals, leaving small cavities in the bone surface. Resorption is followed by the bone formation stage, which is carried out by another set of special cells, called osteoblasts, which fill in the cavities with new bone.

When bone loss outpaces bone formation, the result is low bone mass. When there is less bone, bones become more fragile and are more prone to fracture. Osteoporosis is a disease of severely low bone mass. ■

enter the bone from the blood, is required to keep bones strong.

In the resorption stage of bone remodeling, special cells called osteoclasts invade the surface of the bone and remove both the matrix and minerals, leaving small cavities in the bone surface. This stage is followed by bone formation, which is carried out by another set of special cells, called osteoblasts, which fill in the cavities with new bone. The entire process takes three to six months, which is why broken bones take some time to heal—and why it takes time to assess whether an osteoporosis treatment is working. When the rate of bone loss exceeds the rate of bone formation, the result is low bone mass. Because bone mass is difficult to measure noninvasively, the closely related value of bone mineral density (BMD) is used instead. BMD can be measured with a variety of x-ray techniques.

Bone quality also plays a role in bone strength. Bone quality refers to the overall architecture of bone, which can vary from person to person. Because no noninvasive procedure currently can determine bone quality, measuring BMD is the best way to identify osteoporosis and predict a person's risk of fractures (see "Bone Turnover Biomarkers: Beyond the DXA Scan" on pages 56-57).

Causes of Osteoporosis

The risk of developing osteoporosis increases in both women and men as they grow older. Women are more susceptible than men, because compared with men they have less total bone mass to begin with and because estrogen plays a vital role in bone health. As the production of natural estrogen drops off during menopause, the rate of bone loss begins to pull ahead of the rate of bone formation.

In addition to age and gender, other risk factors include:

- a history of fracture as an adult (especially after age 40)
- a history of fracture in a first-degree relative (male or female)
- ethnicity (white and Asian women are at greater risk than women in other ethnic groups).

Risk factors that *can* be changed include:

- smoking
- low body weight (under 127 lbs for women)
- low estrogen levels in women; low testosterone levels in men
- prolonged low calcium and vitamin D intake
- eating disorders
- lack of exercise (or excessive exercise that leads to missed menstrual periods during a woman's premenopausal years)

- ongoing use of certain drugs, such as corticosteroids like prednisone, or some medications used to treat prostate or breast cancer
- excessive alcohol consumption.

One of the primary determinants of osteoporosis risk is family history. The genes that are important in determining susceptibility to osteoporosis have not been fully identified, but they may account for as much of 70 to 80% of osteoporosis risk.

Osteoporosis also can be caused by other diseases or certain medications. This is called secondary osteoporosis. For instance, many people with severe asthma, rheumatoid arthritis, inflammatory bowel disease, or multiple sclerosis take corticosteroids, which are a common cause of osteoporosis. Other drugs that can cause osteoporosis include anticonvulsants, which are used to treat epilepsy, and inappropriately high doses of thyroid hormone replacement.

Studies have linked a high intake of vitamin A from retinol with increased risk of fractures among men and postmenopausal women, though vitamin A from beta-carotene does not appear to affect risk. Recently, a class of drugs used to treat diabetes, thiazolidinediones, was found to be associated with an increased risk of fracture (see "Osteoporosis and Diabetes: A Dangerous Duo" on pages 50-51).

Certain other hormonal disorders, including an overactive thyroid gland (hyperthyroidism), Cushing's syndrome (excessive steroids produced by the body), and an overactive parathyroid gland (hyperparathyroidism), can cause bone loss in men and women. Inflammatory diseases such as inflammatory bowel disease (Crohn's disease and ulcerative colitis), lupus, and rheumatoid arthritis also can contribute to bone loss, as can malabsorption syndromes such as celiac disease.

If a man develops osteoporosis, a thorough medical evaluation should be performed to determine the underlying cause. Osteoporosis in a premenopausal woman or in any woman who is not responding to treatment also warrants evaluation for secondary causes of the disease.

Complications of Osteoporosis

Osteoporosis is a silent, usually painless, saboteur. For many people, the first sign of trouble is a fracture. But subtle signs may have been present for some time—a gradual loss of height over the years, for instance, the rounding of the upper back (known as kyphosis, or dowager's hump), or even tooth loss.

ASK THE DOCTOR

Q. ***I am a 64-year-old woman who's taking Prilosec for acid reflux. I recently heard that proton pump inhibitors increase the risk of fractures. Should I be worried?***

A. Several studies have linked omeprazole (Prilosec) and other proton pump inhibitors to an increased risk of hip fractures.

The best study to date is a French study published in *Calcified Tissue International* in 2009. In this trial, researchers looked at more than 1,200 postmenopausal women who were participating in the Osteoporosis and Ultrasound Study (OPUS). A total of 5% of the women were taking Prilosec. After six years, the rate of vertebral fractures was significantly higher among women who were using Prilosec than among those who were not: 1.89 per 100 person-years as opposed to 0.60 per 100 person-years.

Researchers can't be certain that the Prilosec caused the increase in fractures; the women taking the drug may have had other conditions (such as infection with *Helicobacter pylori*) that might explain the increase in fractures.

Still, this study raises potential concerns for older women. If you're taking a proton pump inhibitor, ask your doctor whether it's worth switching to a different type of medication. H_2-receptor antagonists appear to be linked to a lower risk of fractures than proton pump inhibitors.

Proton pump inhibitors decrease stomach acid, potentially interfering with absorption of calcium and other nutrients that the bones need.

The most common sites of osteoporosis-related fractures are the spine and hip, but the wrist and other bones may also be affected. Osteoporosis is responsible for more than 2 million fractures a year, including approximately 550,000 spinal (vertebral) fractures, more than 300,000 hip fractures, 400,000 wrist fractures, and 800,000 other fractures.

An expert panel convened by the National Osteoporosis Foundation estimated that at least 90% of all hip and spine fractures in older women are caused by osteoporosis. Anyone who has had one osteoporosis-related fracture is at very high risk for a second.

Some people think that men can't get osteoporosis. That is simply not true. Before age 60, fractures are more common in men than in women, likely because of injuries related to sports and accidents. Although the prevalence of fractures increases in men after age 60, their rate is still less than half that of women of the same age. This is because men enter adulthood with greater bone mass than women—and women rapidly lose bone mass during the first three to five years after a natural or surgical menopause (or any other cause of estrogen deficiency). Nevertheless, one in five men will experience an osteoporosis-related fracture in his lifetime.

The most commonly identified risk factors for osteoporosis in men are excessive alcohol intake, use of corticosteroid drugs (such as prednisone), and hypogonadism (testosterone deficiency).

As mentioned previously, if a man develops osteoporosis, a thorough medical evaluation should be performed to determine the underlying cause. Similarly, a premenopausal woman or any woman who is not responding to treatment should also undergo an evaluation for secondary causes of the disease.

Vertebral Compression Fractures

Compression fractures in people with weakened vertebrae are usually caused either by falling or by placing a load on outstretched arms (for example, by raising a window or lifting a small child or bag of groceries). Such spinal fractures typically cause the front of the vertebrae to collapse.

Bone loss in the spine takes place rapidly around the time of menopause, and estimates suggest that 25% of American women over the age of 50 experience one or more compression fractures of their vertebrae in their lifetime. Men account for approximately one seventh of the vertebral compression fractures associated with osteoporosis.

A vertebral compression fracture due to osteoporosis is accompanied by intense, localized back pain in about 80% of cases, though there may be no pain until a few days after the fracture. When pain does develop, it can be severe enough to incapacitate a person for several weeks. The pain worsens during activities that involve twisting or bending and initially does not ease up, even with bed rest.

Typically, the pain will resolve after several weeks with the use of mild analgesics and rest. The pain may continue and get worse, however, if the bone fails to heal because of a loss of blood supply or if the vertebral deformity that results from the fracture either accelerates degenerative changes in the facet joints or compresses a nerve root.

A frequent problem immediately following a fracture in the lower lumbar region is difficulty with urination and bowel movements. Fortunately, this is temporary.

Longer-term repercussions include stooped posture as well as loss of height. These structural changes reduce the amount of space available for vital organs such as the stomach and lungs. Compression of the stomach causes the abdomen to protrude and creates a sensation of indigestion or fullness that may lead to weight loss, while compression of the chest cavity leads to a reduction in lung capacity that can contribute to breathlessness or lung disease.

Structural changes caused by vertebral compression fractures also weaken the spinal extensor muscles, leading to fatigue. In addition, they can cause concerns about physical appearance and make it difficult to find clothes that fit properly. All of these problems may lead to depression as well as difficulty sitting or sleeping. Rarely, a severe vertebral collapse may cause paralysis by exerting pressure on the spinal cord.

Hip Fractures

Many people fear hip fractures—and with good reason. Of all types of fractures, hip fractures have the most significant impact on the quality of life. Alarmingly, close to 25% of those over age 50 who break a hip will die within a year. In addition, 40% are unable to walk independently a year after they've broken a hip, and 60% are unable to perform basic activities of daily living, such as dressing themselves. Because of these devastating consequences, preserving and boosting bone mass and preventing falls and fractures are crucial.

A hip fracture usually occurs when a person falls from a standing position, with the hip taking the impact of the fall, although less traumatic falls also can cause hip fractures. More than 90% of the 350,000 hip fractures that occur each year in the United States are the result of a fall.

NEW RESEARCH

Major Depression Linked to Low Bone Mineral Density

People who suffer from depression are significantly more likely to have low bone mineral density (BMD), according to a new analysis. The link is especially strong among premenopausal women who have been diagnosed with major depression by a psychiatrist.

Israeli investigators analyzed 23 relevant studies that examined the possible association between depression and skeletal health in a total of 2,327 depressed and 21,141 nondepressed individuals.

The analysis showed that people with depression had significantly lower BMD than those without depression. The link between depression and low BMD was stronger in women than in men, and stronger in premenopausal than in postmenopausal women. Women who had been formally diagnosed by a psychiatrist as having major depression had reductions in BMD, but not those who had been diagnosed with only self-rating questionnaires.

People with depression may be less likely to exercise, which could affect BMD. Antidepressant drugs also have been linked to reductions in BMD, especially selective serotonin reuptake inhibitors.

If you have a history of depression, talk to your doctor about monitoring your BMD. You may need to step up your efforts to prevent or treat osteoporosis.

BIOLOGICAL PSYCHIATRY
Volume 66, page 423
September 1, 2009

Osteoporosis and Diabetes: A Dangerous Duo

Important advice on how to lower your fracture risk

When you think of the possible risk factors for osteoporosis, you probably can name several of the well-recognized ones—like having a family history of fractures or a low body weight or being older, female, or inactive. But what may not immediately come to mind is that certain chronic diseases can interfere with bone health and lead to osteoporosis and fractures.

Scientists now know that one such disease is diabetes. And with an estimated 44 million Americans with osteoporosis or osteopenia (a precursor to osteoporosis) and approximately 24 million with diabetes, the potential public health consequences of this finding are significant.

If you have osteoporosis and diabetes, here's what you need to know to reduce your chances of sustaining a debilitating fracture.

Evidence for a Diabetes-Fracture Link

Numerous studies show a connection between diabetes and bone fractures—particularly hip fractures. Results from the large, 22-year Nurses' Health Study found that women with type 1 diabetes were six times more likely than women without diabetes to have a hip fracture. Women with type 2 diabetes had more than twice the risk. Even after controlling for factors that increase the chances of both fractures and diabetes, such as age, body weight, and physical activity, the elevated risk remained.

Men are at increased risk as well, according to a recent review of 16 studies, published in the *American Journal of Epidemiology*. After reviewing the records of more than 800,000 men and women, the researchers found that those with type 1 diabetes were six times more likely to experience a hip fracture than those who didn't have diabetes, and people with type 2 diabetes were nearly twice as likely. On average, men with diabetes had a slightly greater risk of hip fractures than women with diabetes.

Explaining the Link

A logical explanation is that people with diabetes have lower bone mineral density (BMD) than people without diabetes. And research shows that this is true for people with type 1 disease and that the hormone insulin may play a role.

Type 1 diabetes occurs when the body destroys it own pancreas; This leads to a deficiency of insulin, which is essential in promoting bone strength and growth and helping children and young adults achieve their peak bone mass. What's more, type 1 diabetes typically develops before age 30—the time when most people are building bone to reach their peak bone mass.

But a lack of insulin is only one of the factors contributing to an increased risk of fractures in individuals with type 1 diabetes. In addition, it doesn't explain the increased fracture risk in those with type 2 disease, who tend to have normal or elevated BMD and to be overweight, both of which help protect against fractures. Also, type 2 diabetes usually arises in middle age and is mostly related to decreased insulin sensitivity rather than reduced insulin production. So investigators have proposed several other possibilities.

Blood glucose levels. People with poorly controlled diabetes have high blood glucose levels (hyperglycemia), which may directly affect bone quality—an indicator of bone strength not measured by a BMD test. High blood glucose levels also increase your risk of diabetes complications, many of which raise the likelihood of falls and fractures (see below).

Conversely, people who take diabetes medication, particularly insulin, are at risk for hypoglycemia (low blood glucose levels) when they do not closely match drug doses to food intake and physical activity. Symptoms of hypoglycemia like dizziness, lack of coordination, and muscle weakness can increase your risk of falls and thus fractures.

Diabetes complications. People with diabetes are at high risk for a range of complications, including eye disease, nerve problems, cardiovascular disease, and kidney dysfunction. Eye problems like diabetic retinopathy, cataracts, and glaucoma can impair vision, increasing the chances of falls. Nerve problems, especially those in the feet and legs, can negatively affect balance and make falls more likely. Cardiovascular disease causes plaque buildup and narrowing of the arteries, which may decrease blood flow to the bones and, like high blood glucose levels, have a detrimental effect on bone quality. Last, people with diabetes-related kidney disease may not absorb enough vitamin D, which is essential for calcium absorption and bone health.

Medications. A class of drugs known as thiazolidinediones, used to treat type 2 diabetes, may be a culprit, too. A recent review of 12 studies—including 10 randomized, controlled trials and more than 45,000 people—found that women with type 2 diabetes who used thiazolidinediones for a year or more had twice the risk of fracture as nonusers. Another recent study of nearly 5,000 people, reported in the *Archives of Internal Medicine*, found that both men and women who used thiazolidinediones for more than a year were twice as likely to have a fracture, particularly of the hip or wrist, than nonusers.

Researchers believe that thiazolidinediones cause bone marrow stem cells to become adipocytes (fat cells) rather than osteoblasts (cells responsible for bone formation), thereby weakening the bones.

Two thiazolidinediones, rosiglitazone (Avandia) and pioglitazone (Actos), are approved in the United States. Combination products containing rosiglitazone (Avandaryl, Avandamet) and pioglitazone (Actoplus Met, Duetact) also are available.

Shared risk factors. Older age and a sedentary lifestyle are risk factors for type 2 diabetes and fractures. So it's possible that the link between these two health problems may simply be that they share a risk factor or two. However, when studies control for these risk factors, the relationship between type 2 diabetes and fractures holds true.

Lower Your Fracture Risk

If you have diabetes, the following steps can help reduce your risk of sustaining a debilitating fracture.

See your ophthalmologist regularly. Vision problems can increase your risk of falling and sustaining a fracture. Be sure to see your eye doctor for a check-up every six to 12 months, take your eye medication as prescribed, and call your doctor right away if you develop vision problems between regularly scheduled visits.

Control your glucose levels. Episodes of hypoglycemia (low blood sugar level) or hyperglycemia (high blood sugar level) can raise your risk of diabetes complications as well as falls and fractures. To lower the risks, carefully follow your doctor's advice on diet and exercise, take your medications as prescribed, routinely check your blood glucose levels at home, and aim for an A1c level of around 7%. Your doctor should measure your A1c levels with a blood test every three to six months. The test is an indicator of your average blood glucose level over the past few months.

Pay attention to your calcium and vitamin D intake. To strengthen your bones, be sure you're consuming enough calcium and vitamin D. The National Osteoporosis Foundation recommends 1,000 mg of calcium and 400 to 800 IU of vitamin D a day for men and women under age 50. If you are 50 or older, you should try to consume 1,200 mg of calcium and 800 to 1,000 IU of vitamin D daily. You may need to take supplements to reach these levels.

Get moving. Exercise is a win-win situation for people with diabetes and osteoporosis. It can help reduce blood glucose levels and increase your bone strength. Aim for at least 30 minutes of low-impact, weight-bearing exercises like walking or low-impact aerobics on most—and preferably all—days of the week. Also, be sure to incorporate activities into your exercise routine that help develop muscle strength and improve balance.

Before starting a new exercise regimen, always check with your doctor first for any restrictions or any dietary or medication modifications you will need to make. If you're not sure how to get started, ask your doctor to refer you to a physical therapist who can develop an exercise regimen that meets your osteoporosis and diabetes needs.

Stop smoking. Smoking is a known risk factor for hip fractures in women and men, and studies show that smoking cessation can reduce your risk. If you're having difficulty quitting, talk to your doctor about the nicotine replacement products, prescription drugs, and counseling programs that can significantly increase your odds of success.

Review your medications. If you are taking a thiazolidinedione, particularly if you have other risk factors for osteoporosis, ask your doctor if there is another medication—for example, metformin (Fortamet, Glucophage, Glumetza) or a sulfonylurea like glyburide (DiaBeta, Glynase, Micronase)—that can control your diabetes. If you continue taking a thiazolidinedione, ask your doctor to evaluate your other risk factors for a fracture and whether you should have more frequent BMD tests and take additional aggressive measures to safeguard the health of your bones. ■

The rate of hip fracture begins to increase at age 50, doubling every five to six years. Nearly half of the women who reach age 90 have had a hip fracture. Men account for nearly 30% of hip fractures.

The risk factors for a hip fracture are:

- being older than 65
- being female
- having a family history of fractures later in life
- low body weight
- poor nutrition
- smoking or excessive alcohol use
- mental impairment
- poor eyesight
- unsteady balance
- frailty.

The symptoms of hip fracture are not subtle. They include pain in the groin or buttock, inability to put weight on the leg on the affected side, or pain when trying to bear weight. Hip fractures may also interrupt the nerves or blood vessels that supply the leg.

All hip fractures require surgical repair or replacement, and treatment is often required for injuries related to the fall, such as head injuries.

Other Osteoporotic Fractures

Because osteoporosis affects bone mass throughout the skeleton, it can lead to fractures anywhere in the body. Both the type and location of the trauma usually determine the kind of fracture that is involved. For example, falling on an outstretched hand can lead to a specific type of wrist and forearm injury known as a Colles' fracture (a break at the end of one of the bones in the forearm). The wrist, toes, and ribs are among the most common sites of osteoporotic fractures. For an individual with severe osteoporosis, simply sneezing or coughing may be enough to cause painful fractures of the ribs and spine. Such fractures can sometimes lead to deformities as well as pain.

Diagnosing Osteoporosis

The National Osteoporosis Foundation recommends that all women age 65 and older get screened for osteoporosis. In addition, postmenopausal women who are under age 65 but have additional risk factors for osteoporosis (such as use of corticosteroids or a family history of osteoporosis) or who have recently had a fracture should be screened. Although widespread screening of premenopausal and perimenopausal women is not generally recommended, it might be appropriate depending on your individual health profile.

An individualized approach to screening based on advancing age and risk factor profile is optimal. For instance, if you are a perimenopausal woman in your early 50s with several significant risk factors, such as smoking, low body weight, and white ethnicity, your doctor may feel that testing is warranted.

The National Osteoporosis Foundation also recommends that all men age 70 and older be screened for osteoporosis. Men who are between the ages of 50 and 70 should be tested for osteoporosis if they are at high risk. Men may be at high risk if they:

- take a hormone-blocking drug for prostate cancer such as leuprolide (Lupron)
- smoke
- drink too much alcohol (three or more drinks per day)
- take steroids to treat diseases such as rheumatoid arthritis or asthma
- have a chronic disease that affects the lungs, kidneys, stomach, or intestines or alters hormone levels
- have a low testosterone level
- don't consume enough calcium or vitamin D
- don't get enough exercise.

Your doctor may use a new electronic tool called FRAX, which stands for fracture risk assessment tool, to give you an assessment of your fracture risk based on your individual profile.

Medical History and Physical Examination

During an osteoporosis examination, the doctor will take an inventory of risk factors, including family history, history of fractures, menstrual history, dietary history, medications, habits such as cigarette smoking and alcohol consumption, and a review of past illnesses. The physical exam includes an assessment of spinal tenderness and curvature, height measurement, and a search for signs of other medical conditions that may contribute to osteoporosis.

Laboratory Tests

In select cases, blood and urine tests may be required to evaluate for medical conditions that can lead to osteoporosis. Blood tests include those that measure levels of calcium, thyroid-stimulating hormone, parathyroid hormone, the enzyme alkaline phosphatase, and vitamin D, as well as kidney and liver function tests. Calcium and cortisol may be measured in the urine.

When active bone resorption occurs in people with osteoporosis or Paget's disease, the urine shows increased amounts of collagen byproducts—pyridinium cross-links and N-telopeptides—created by the breakdown of bone. Urine tests for these substances (such as Osteomark) have been approved by the FDA and are commercially available, but their usefulness is not universally accepted. For more information, see "Bone Turnover Biomarkers: Beyond the DXA Scan" on pages 56-57.

Although tests for pyridinium cross-links and N-telopeptides are not required for a diagnosis of osteoporosis, they are useful in assessing a person's response to therapy, because they can gauge response after just a few months of treatment. By comparison, it takes much longer to assess response to therapy using x-ray tests such as DXA scans, which generally are not repeated until you have completed a full year of treatment.

Bone Mineral Density Tests

Bone mineral density (BMD) tests are performed in individuals who are at risk for osteoporosis or have experienced a suspicious fracture. These tests help doctors diagnose osteoporosis or osteopenia (low bone mass, a warning sign for osteoporosis). BMD tests can also predict a person's risk of experiencing a fracture, monitor progression of bone loss over time, and observe how well osteoporosis treatments are working.

To measure BMD, your doctor can use a variety of techniques. Generally, these fall into two categories: tests that measure BMD in the central areas of the body (that is, the spine, hip, and total body) and those that measure BMD in peripheral areas (for example, the wrist, finger, shinbone, kneecap, and heel).

All of the BMD tests are painless and safe. While the central techniques are considered the most precise, they are more expensive than the peripheral tests. In addition, the equipment used for the test is not portable. The type of test your doctor performs may reflect a balance between your needs and the availability of BMD equipment in your area.

After starting treatment, you may undergo BMD testing at one year to monitor your response to therapy. After this point, retesting every two to three years is recommended. Your doctor may want you to be retested more often if you're switching from one treatment to another or you continue to experience rapid bone loss.

Central techniques

Central BMD tests include dual-energy x-ray absorptiometry and quantitative computed tomography. (Dual-photon absorptiometry, an older test, is used only rarely today.)

Dual-energy x-ray absorptiometry (DXA). This technique is the "gold standard" for the measurement of BMD. As the name implies, it involves the use of two x-ray beams aimed at the bone. A computer analyzes the amount of energy that passes through the bone and uses the measurement to calculate BMD. The test takes about 20 minutes and involves a low radiation exposure.

DXA is a valuable test for monitoring BMD changes over time as well as a person's response to osteoporosis treatment. Although DXA is the best tool for measuring BMD, it doesn't provide accurate spinal measurements in people with a spinal deformity, arthritis in the lower spine, or a history of spinal surgery. Also, hip measurements are not accurate in a hip that has been replaced or contains metal hardware.

BMD results from DXA are given as a T-score, which reflects how much the BMD is above or below normal. In general, a T-score of -1.0 or higher is considered to be normal, and a T-score of -2.5 or lower indicates osteoporosis. A person with a score between -1.0 and -2.5 may eventually develop osteoporosis or be at risk for a future fracture. A score in this range is considered osteopenia.

Quantitative computed tomography (QCT). This procedure is not well studied or standardized, but it is sometimes performed instead of DXA to analyze bone density in the spine. QCT is similar to a regular computed tomography (CT) scan, in which x-rays generate a series of cross-sectional pictures that create a three-dimensional image. QCT simply uses different software than standard CT to analyze BMD. It takes about 10 to 15 minutes to perform, exposes the body to more radiation than other central or peripheral bone measurement methods (including DXA), and generally costs more than DXA.

Peripheral techniques

Peripheral techniques used to measure BMD include quantitative ultrasound, peripheral dual-energy x-ray absorptiometry, radiographic absorptiometry, peripheral quantitative computed tomography, and single-energy x-ray absorptiometry. Quantitative ultrasound and peripheral dual-energy x-ray absorptiometry are the most widely used. (Single-photon absorptiometry, an older test, is rarely used.)

Peripheral techniques are valuable for osteoporosis screening; however, their lack of precision makes them less useful for following changes in BMD over time or for tracking response to therapy. In

ASK THE DOCTOR

Q. ***My doctor recommended that I start eating a low-fat diet to reduce my risk of heart disease now that I've gone through menopause. Will changing the way I eat affect my bones?***

A. It's true that losing a lot of weight by dieting when you're older can weaken your bones, which is an extra reason to get plenty of exercise as part of a weight loss plan. But switching to a low-fat diet seems to be safe for your bones, according to a new study.

In the Women's Health Initiative Dietary Modification Trial, published in the *American Journal of Clinical Nutrition* in 2009, researchers randomly assigned close to 49,000 postmenopausal women to either a low-fat diet or their regular diet. The low-fat diet limited fat to 20% of daily calories and was rich in fruit, vegetables, and whole grains.

After an average of eight years, the risk of osteoporotic fractures was no different between the two groups—even though there was a small decrease in bone mineral density at the hip among people in the low-fat diet group.

So go ahead and follow the diet that your doctor is recommending. To be sure you're getting plenty of calcium and vitamin D, don't cut back on dairy. Instead, substitute low-fat for full-fat dairy.

Bone Turnover Biomarkers: Beyond the DXA Scan

Can a simple blood or urine test identify people at risk for osteoporosis?

Biomarker—A biological molecule found in blood, other body fluids, or tissues that is a sign of a normal or abnormal process or of a condition or disease. A biomarker may be used to see how well the body responds to treatment for a disease or condition.

Wondering what a biomarker is? One of the most well-known examples is prostate-specific antigen, or PSA, a protein that is made and excreted only by the prostate. Using a simple blood test, doctors can measure the level of PSA in a man's bloodstream. An elevated level alerts the doctor to the possibility of prostate cancer. PSA tests are also used to monitor response to prostate cancer treatment and to determine if the disease is progressing.

In a similar vein, researchers are investigating bone-related biomarkers as a tool to identify people with or at risk for osteoporosis, to monitor response to osteoporosis treatment, and to assess the future risk of fractures. Here's an update on the latest findings.

A Brief Lesson on Bone Turnover

Bone remodeling, also known as turnover, is a continuous process by which old bone is removed and new bone is added. The two stages of bone remodeling—resorption and formation—involve the activity of special cells called osteoclasts (cells that resorb old bone) and osteoblasts (cells that form new bone). Usually, the amount of bone being resorbed is equal to the amount being formed and the bone mass remains constant. But when bone resorption starts to occur more quickly than bone formation, which happens in many postmenopausal women, it can lead to osteoporosis and, potentially, an increased risk of fractures.

Known Markers of Bone Turnover

During the bone remodeling process, the osteoblasts and osteoclasts produce enzymes and other proteins that are released into the bloodstream and eventually excreted in the urine. These compounds, or biomarkers, are divided into two main categories: markers of bone resorption and markers of bone formation.

Researchers have identified several of these biomarkers. For example, N-terminal type I collagen telopeptide (NTX), C-terminal type I collagen telopeptide (CTX), deoxypyridinoline (DPD), hydroxyproline, and tartrate-resistent acid phosphatase (TRAP) are all markers of bone resorption. NTX, DPD, and hydroxyproline can be measured in urine; TRAP, in blood; and CTX in blood and urine.

Bone formation biomarkers include procollagen I N-terminal extension propeptide (PINP), bone-specific alkaline phosphatase (BSAP), osteocalcin (OCN), and procollagen I C-terminal extension propeptide (PICP). These biomarkers can be measured in the blood.

Diagnosing Osteoporosis

If you have a high level of one of the bone resorption markers mentioned above, it could be a sign of bone loss and thus osteoporosis. However, bone turnover biomarkers won't likely replace bone mineral density (BMD) testing as the standard method of diagnosing osteoporosis.

The reason? Not one bone

addition, peripheral techniques cannot measure hip or spine BMD; the sites where fractures have the most serious consequences.

Quantitative ultrasound (QUS)

This technique involves passing high-frequency sound waves through bone to measure its density in peripheral sites like the shinbone, heel, turnover marker has shown sufficient sensitivity or specificity for diagnosing osteoporosis. A sensitive test is good at not missing a person who has the condition; a specific test does well at not accidentally labeling a person with a medical condition that he or she doesn't have.

Researchers are still on the hunt for biomarkers with better sensitivity and specificity. Still, elevated levels of bone turnover markers are possible signs of disease, just like high levels of PSA are. In the case of PSA, the disease is prostate cancer; for bone turnover markers, the disease is osteoporosis. But a diagnosis cannot be made on the presence of these biomarkers alone. Further testing—a prostate biopsy or a BMD test such as a DXA scan, respectively—is still required.

Monitoring Therapy

Bone turnover markers are probably most valuable as a method of monitoring response to osteoporosis therapy.

Research shows that significant changes in levels of bone-turnover biomarkers are observed three to six months following the initiation of therapy. By comparison, meaningful changes in BMD can't be detected by DXA scan until 12 to 24 months after treatment starts.

Thus, use of bone turnover biomarkers could help your doctor determine in a more timely manner whether your treatment is working or needs to be modified. When effective, antiresorptive therapies like bisphophonates or raloxifene (Evista) produce reductions in markers of bone resorption, whereas anabolic therapies, such as teriparatide (Forteo), result in increases in markers of bone formation and bone resorption indicative of increased bone remodeling.

Assessing Fracture Risk

Bone mineral density testing cannot be used alone to predict future fracture risk. In addition to your T-score (which reflects how much your BMD is above or below normal), doctors must consider such factors as your age, gender, weight, and nutritional status. Bone turnover biomarkers are yet another possible factor doctors could add to the mix.

One large investigation, the Epidemiology of Osteoporosis (EPIDOS) study, which involved nearly 7,600 healthy women older than age 75, found that certain markers of bone turnover (CTX, DPD, and osteocalcin) were higher in women who had sustained a hip fracture than in those who remained fracture free over a two-year period. Other research shows that high NTX, BSAP, and TRAP levels in women also are associated with an increased risk of fracture.

Although there is less information on men, the six-year Dubbo Osteoporosis Epidemiology Study (DOES) found that increased levels of the bone resorption marker carboxyterminal telopeptide of type 1 collagen (ICTP) were associated with an increased risk of fracture in elderly males.

Studies also show that using the results of both BMD and biomarker tests improves the ability to predict future fractures, suggesting that levels of bone turnover markers provide additional risk information not measured by the standard BMD test.

Coming to Your Doctor's Office Soon?

More research is needed before the use of bone turnover biomarkers becomes as routine as PSA testing. But stay tuned. Many experts believe that biomarkers will, in due course, play an important role in osteoporosis management—particularly when used as a complement to BMD testing to determine who's most at risk for fractures and to evaluate treatment effectiveness. ■

and kneecap. There is no exposure to radiation, and screening takes less than five minutes. Research indicates that QUS may be as accurate as DXA in predicting fracture risk and diagnosing osteoporosis.

Peripheral dual-energy x-ray absorptiometry (pDXA)

This test is similar to a central DXA test except that it uses a portable machine and measures BMD in the finger, wrist, or heel. It takes less than five minutes to perform, and exposure to radiation is low.

Radiographic absorptiometry (RA)
This test uses regular x-ray technology to determine BMD in the hand. The x-ray is taken with a "reference wedge" placed near the hand; this wedge has a known density with which the density of bone in the hand is then compared. In general, the results of RA testing provide an accurate measure of bone density. RA takes just one to three minutes to perform, and the test involves only a small exposure to radiation.

Peripheral quantitative computed tomography (pQCT)
pQCT is similar to the central QCT scan, except that it is used to measure BMD in the wrist. The scan takes about 10 minutes, and the results are generally accurate. Peripheral QCT is less expensive than central QCT, and exposure to radiation is lower.

Single-energy x-ray absorptiometry (SXA)
This test is commonly used to determine BMD in the heel or wrist. The procedure is similar in principle to DXA, except that it uses one x-ray beam instead of two. SXA takes about 10 to 15 minutes, and the exposure to radiation is minimal.

Preventing Osteoporosis

Osteoporosis prevention relies on a three-pronged approach of exercise, proper nutrition, and—when appropriate—medication, including some bisphosphonates (see Bisphosphonates on pages 64-65). While women are more likely than men to develop osteoporosis, men, too, should get regular exercise, eat well, and minimize other risk factors.

Exercise

Exercise is an important component of osteoporosis prevention. The more active you are, the stronger your bones will be. Certain types of exercise are more beneficial than others for preventing osteoporosis. Your exercise routine should include weight-bearing and resistance exercises and ideally should begin well before menopause. Older people should incorporate balance exercises into their routine (see "Start Your Engines!" on pages 60-61).

Nutrition

Although calcium is in the nutritional spotlight for its role in preventing osteoporosis, vitamin D also is essential. A number of other nutrients provided by a well-rounded, healthy diet play a role in building healthy bone as well.

Calcium

For men and women age 19 to 50, the recommended daily intake (Dietary Reference Intake, or DRI) for calcium is 1,000 mg per day. After age 50, the DRI increases to 1,200 mg per day.

The best sources of calcium are low-fat milk and other dairy products. For example, one cup of milk contains 300 mg of calcium, and one cup of plain, low-fat yogurt contains 415 mg. Low-fat dairy products contain slightly more calcium than their full-fat counterparts—low-fat milk actually contains slightly more than 300 mg of calcium per cup, while full-fat milk contains slightly less. But the real reason to choose low-fat products is to avoid excessive intake of saturated fat.

If you have lactose intolerance (an inability to digest the naturally occurring sugars in milk) and dairy foods give you digestive problems, you will need to include other sources of calcium in your diet such as canned salmon with bones (3 oz contains 200 mg of calcium), leafy green vegetables, almonds, calcium-fortified cereals, and calcium-fortified orange juice.

Despite these dietary sources of calcium, surveys show that most people get less than the DRI for calcium from their diet. In fact, a dietary intake of only 400 mg of calcium per day is quite common. Although meeting the DRI is possible with careful dietary planning, most people need to take daily supplements that provide an additional 500 to 1,000 mg of calcium.

A variety of calcium supplements are available. Calcium carbonate and calcium citrate contain the highest percentage of calcium in each tablet, but calcium citrate is more readily absorbed from the intestine. You should take calcium carbonate pills with meals because this type of calcium is absorbed better in the presence of stomach acid.

Vitamin D

Many people neglect to take a proper amount of vitamin D. A recent study found that women with low blood levels of vitamin D were at increased risk for hip fracture. Without vitamin D, the body cannot absorb calcium properly.

NEW RESEARCH

Exercise Reverses Bone Loss Caused By Weight Loss

Weight loss has one health disadvantage: a reduction in bone mineral density (BMD). But a new study finds that adding exercise to a weight loss program can actually increase BMD, possibly by reducing inflammation.

The study included 86 overweight or obese postmenopausal women who participated in a weight loss program, either on its own or combined with walking three days a week for 45 to 60 minutes.

Six months later, women in both groups had lost weight. BMD at the femoral neck (part of the hip joint) increased by about 2% for women in the weight loss plus walking program but did not change for those in the weight loss-only program. Women in the exercise group also had increases in aerobic capacity and reductions in markers of inflammation, such as tumor necrosis factor and interleukin; these improvements didn't occur in the other group. The researchers theorized that exercise may halt the bone resorption that can occur during weight loss by reducing inflammation in the body.

Although dieting is effective on its own for weight loss, you still need exercise to keep your bones strong.

CALCIFIED TISSUE INTERNATIONAL
Volume 84, page 257
April 2009

Start Your Engines!

Preserve your bone health with a three-pronged exercise plan

Your body is one remarkable machine, but it needs regular physical activity to help keep itself tuned. If you have osteoporosis or are at risk for it, a well-balanced exercise routine can improve your bone health and decrease your risk of falling.

Your best bet: a combination exercise program that includes weight-bearing aerobic exercise, resistance training, and balance exercises. This sounds like a tall order, but you can achieve meaningful improvement in your bone health if you perform the right exercises regularly.

The Case for a Combination Program

Beginning an exercise program is never easy, and rather than doing nothing, many of us think, "I'll at least start walking. I can handle that. Besides, it's good for my heart, too." But when it comes to improving your bone health, a growing body of evidence demonstrates that a regular stroll—or even a brisk walk—may not be enough.

British researchers recently reviewed eight studies that looked at whether walking was beneficial in preserving bone mineral density (BMD) among postmenopausal women. Their findings, reported in the journal *Bone*, showed that participating in a regular walking regimen for six months to two years failed to preserve spine BMD. However, regular walking did preserve BMD at the femoral neck (part of the thigh bone that connects to the hip joint).

What Else Should You Do?

Osteoporosis experts recommend a three-pronged program consisting of weight-bearing aerobic exercise, resistance training, and balance exercises. Walking can still be part of your exercise routine, but it needs to be done along with muscle strengthening and balance training to make a difference in your risk of bone loss and falls.

Weight-bearing aerobic exercise. The bones in your lower spine, hips, and legs bear all of your body mass during weight-bearing exercise. This stress on your bones and the pull of attached muscles work against gravity and promote bone formation, helping to increase bone density.

Walking, jogging, hiking, dancing, stair climbing, aerobics, and tennis are all examples of weight-bearing exercises. High-impact weight-bearing exercise, such as jogging and aerobics, may be appropriate for those with mildly reduced bone density or osteopenia. However, if you have osteoporosis, it's safer to perform weight-bearing exercises that have less impact on your bones. Examples include walking, elliptical training, stair step machines, and low-impact aerobics.

For best results, shoot for 30 minutes a day of weight-bearing activities on five to seven days a week.

Resistance training. Resistance exercises, also known as strength or muscle-building exercises, involve lifting your own body weight (calisthenics), lifting free weights, or using weight machines or resistance bands. With this training, you're applying resistance to a specific set of muscles and bones to strengthen them.

Resistance training is particularly helpful for building strength and slowing bone loss in the back and arms, areas of the body that do not benefit from weight-bearing aerobic exercise. Calisthenics, light dumbbells, and resistance bands are the safest ways to build muscle strength for people who have osteoporosis.

You should aim to do resistance training two or three days a week with a day's rest in between to allow your muscles to recover. For a sample resistance-training routine, go to www.nia.nih.gov/HealthInformation/Publications/ExerciseGuide or call 800-222-2225 and ask for a print copy of *Exercise & Physical Activity: Your Everyday Guide from the National Institute on Aging*.

Balance exercises. Although osteoporosis is an important and well-recognized risk factor for bone fractures, so, too, is a recent fall. You can reduce your risk of falls with weight-bearing exercise and resistance training, but exercises that specifically improve balance are helpful, too.

A simple balance exercise is to stand behind a chair and hold onto it with one hand while you raise one leg several inches off the ground. Hold for a count of 10 seconds, and repeat with the other leg. Once you learn to maintain your balance in this position, try holding onto the chair with one fingertip. When you master that, try it without holding on.

Another option is tai chi. According to a report in the *Journal of the American Geriatrics Society*, a randomized, controlled trial involving more than 700 seniors found that 16 weekly sessions of tai chi for one hour improved balance and significantly reduced the risk of falling. Walking also can help with balance, but be careful. Slippery leaves, loose rocks, and uneven sidewalks can be hazards. It is safest to walk on well-lit, well-tended trails or other paths that have minimal irregularities.

Balance exercises can be performed daily. For a sample balance routine, go to the National Institute of Aging website mentioned on the opposite page.

The Keys to Success

Sticking with a well-rounded exercise program will serve you well—for your bones and your whole being. To stay motivated, choose exercises that pique your interest and are within your comfort zone.

Also consider exercising with a friend or family member, or check with your local community center or hospital to see if they offer classes or exercise programs for people with osteoporosis. Your local chapter of the Arthritis Foundation may have appropriate classes as well; they are not just for people with arthritis. ■

Exercise Prudence—Six Safety Tips for People With Osteoporosis

If you have osteoporosis or a previous fragility fracture, here are six safety-related exercise tips to keep in mind:

1. Check with your doctor before starting a new exercise routine. He or she may want you to undergo a bone density test and fitness evaluation to determine the exercises that are beneficial and safe based on your fracture risk, age, medical history, and physical condition. Also ask whether any medications you're taking may affect your alertness, coordination, and balance, which could increase your risk of falls during exercise. Knowing that your exercise program is personalized to your individual health status, fitness abilities, and exercise needs can help ease any fears you may have about starting.
2. Consult your doctor about the appropriateness of high-impact exercises, such as jogging, running, or jumping. These activities can stress the spine, hips, and legs and lead to fractures in people with osteoporosis. Lower-impact exercises like walking or tai chi, which involve slower, controlled movements are much safer. Also avoid exercises with the potential for serious falls, like ice-skating or skiing. Other activities that may be risky in those with severe osteoporosis include bowling and golf.
3. If you have or are at high risk for vertebral compression fractures, avoid movements that twist, flex, or bend your spine (like toe touches, sit-ups, rowing, golf, tennis, and some yoga moves). Moving in these ways can cause undue stress on your vertebrae, increasing your risk of a spinal fracture. Heavy lifting can be harmful as well.
4. If your muscles are sore for more than two days, ease up on your exercise routine and increase your activity level in a more gradual way. Always stop your exercise and consult your doctor if you feel unusual pain or discomfort.
5. Consider enlisting the help of a physical therapist, who can develop a safe exercise plan for you and show you how to correctly perform the exercises and slowly increase their difficulty over time. To find a physical therapist, ask your doctor for a referral or search the directory of the American Physical Therapy Association. To access the directory, go to www.apta.org and click on the "Find a PT" link. Choosing an expertise like Geriatrics, Orthopedics, or Women's Health should help narrow your search to a physical therapist who has experience working with people with osteoporosis.
6. Be extra cautious if you have had a previous fall or fracture or are frail. Your doctor or physical therapist will advise you on how to proceed safely.

A number of studies have confirmed that vitamin D intake helps prevent osteoporosis and lower the risk of fractures in older adults. Vitamin D not only helps with the absorption of calcium, but also aids in the biochemical process by which calcium turns into bone.

Most vitamin D is synthesized by the skin in response to sunlight. In nature, very few foods contain vitamin D. While some foods are fortified—especially breakfast cereals and milk products—studies have shown that the amount listed on the label does not always reflect the contents accurately.

The National Osteoporosis Foundation recommends that women and men under age 50 consume 400 to 800 IU of vitamin D per day. For people age 50 and over, 800 to 1,000 IU daily is recommended.

Other nutrients

A healthy diet rich in fruits and vegetables will provide plenty of phosphorus, magnesium, and vitamins C and K, all of which play a role in bone health.

Vitamin A caution

If you take a daily multivitamin, choose one that contains no more than 900 micrograms (mcg) of vitamin A for men and 700 mcg for women. Also make sure that at least 20% of its vitamin A is in the form of beta-carotene. As mentioned earlier, research suggests that a high intake of vitamin A from retinol might increase the risk of hip fractures in postmenopausal women; too much vitamin A has also been associated with fractures in men.

Hormone Replacement Therapy (HRT)

Among its many other effects on the female body, the hormone estrogen stimulates the bone-building ability of osteoblasts and suppresses the bone-destroying activity of osteoclasts. At menopause, when estrogen levels fall, women suddenly experience a rapid loss of bone and an increased risk of fractures.

Hormone replacement therapy (HRT) involves taking estrogen to treat menopausal symptoms, such as hot flashes, night sweats, and vaginal dryness. The most common HRT formulation also contains a synthetic form of progesterone to counteract the increased risk of uterine cancer in women who take estrogen alone. Women who have had a hysterectomy are able to take estrogen without progesterone.

In addition to easing the symptoms of menopause, HRT reduces the rapid loss of bone that accompanies it. The sooner HRT begins after menopause, the greater the preservation of bone.

However, the decision to use HRT should not be taken lightly. One of the most common forms of HRT, conjugated equine estrogen plus medroxyprogesterone (Prempro), has been found to increase the risk of breast cancer and cardiovascular events (such as heart attacks, strokes, and blood clots) when taken for several years. For this reason, women should not take HRT for any longer than needed to treat menopausal symptoms.

If a woman is concerned about bone loss and thinking about HRT, she should discuss her personal risk and benefit profile with her doctor. Despite the fact that HRT continues to be recommended for preventing osteoporosis, other drugs are available that can accomplish the same goal.

One final note: As soon as HRT is discontinued, bone loss will begin again. Thus it is important to assess the need for osteoporosis treatment before discontinuing HRT.

Testosterone in men

Men with abnormally low levels of testosterone, which can cause osteoporosis, can take testosterone replacement therapy to help preserve their bones. For more information, see Treatment in Men on pages 71-72.

Corticosteroid Caution

Because the prolonged use of corticosteroids such as prednisone can result in significant reductions in bone mass, the American College of Rheumatology (ACR) has issued guidelines for preventing osteoporosis in people taking corticosteroids for longer than six months (typically individuals with such disorders as severe asthma, rheumatoid arthritis, inflammatory bowel disease, or multiple sclerosis). Because prednisone dosages as low as 7.5 mg per day can result in bone loss and an increased risk of fractures, the lowest effective dose should always be used. Corticosteroid formulations that are applied to the skin or inhaled cause fewer side effects than those taken orally.

The guidelines suggest getting a BMD measurement when beginning steroid therapy (or as soon as possible thereafter), following the lifestyle recommendations, and possibly using one of the preventive medications discussed on pages 64-65. Two bisphosphonates that have been approved by the FDA for the prevention of steroid-induced osteoporosis are alendronate (Fosamax) and risedronate (Actonel). In addition, the ACR guidelines suggest taking extra calcium—a total of 1,500 mg a day—and 800 IU of vitamin D.

NEW RESEARCH

Fortified Ice Cream Can Boost Calcium Levels

Fortified ice cream may be a useful strategy to add calcium to your diet, a new study suggests. Results show that calcium absorption from calcium-enriched ice cream is as good as the absorption from milk.

For the study, 16 healthy adults ate a standard breakfast on three separate test days along with ice cream or milk. The ice cream contained either a low level of butterfat (3%) or a typical level of coconut oil (9%) and was fortified with calcium. The reduced-fat milk contained 1.7% milk fat. Blood samples from the volunteers were used to measure calcium absorption.

The difference in calcium absorption among the three groups was not considered statistically significant: 26% for the reduced-butterfat ice cream, 28% for the regular coconut-oil ice cream, and 31% for the reduced-fat milk.

Although fortified ice cream could provide an attractive way to boost your calcium intake, it contains more sugars and fats than milk does. So concentrate on getting calcium from foods like low-fat milk and yogurt, and consider adding calcium-fortified orange juice and soy beverages if your intake is still low. Save the calcium-enriched ice cream, if it becomes available, for an occasional treat.

JOURNAL OF THE AMERICAN DIETETIC ASSOCIATION
Volume 109, page 812
May 2009

Treating Osteoporosis

Treatment of osteoporosis starts with the same three-pronged plan used for prevention: exercise (see page 58), nutrition (see page 59), and medication.

Medication

Medications approved for treating osteoporosis fall into the following general categories: bisphosphonates, selective estrogen receptor modulators, hormone and hormone-like preparations, and anabolic agents. (The chart on pages 66-69 gives an overview of drugs approved for osteoporosis treatment.)

Bisphosphonates

The bisphosphonates are the drugs most often prescribed to treat and prevent osteoporosis. Bisphosphonates help to preserve bone mass by slowing down bone resorption. Clinical studies of these drugs have focused on their effect on BMD and fracture risk.

Members of this drug class include Fosamax, ibandronate (Boniva), Actonel, and zoledronic acid (Reclast). Fosamax and Actonel are indicated for the treatment of postmenopausal osteoporosis in women, for corticosteroid-induced osteoporosis in both women and men, and for other types of osteoporosis in men. Boniva and Reclast are indicated for the treatment of osteoporosis in postmenopausal women.

As mentioned previously, Fosamax and Actonel are also approved for the prevention of osteoporosis.

Although not approved for treating osteoporosis, three other bisphosphonates—etidronate (Didronel), pamidronate (Aredia), and tiludronate (Skelid)—are used for this purpose.

Combined estrogen replacement and bisphosphonate therapies have a modest additive effect in boosting bone mass. Several trials have shown that women with existing osteoporosis have a greater increase in BMD when treated with combination therapy than with either drug therapy alone.

Oral bisphosphonates are not easily absorbed, and they may lead to gastrointestinal side effects such as indigestion, diarrhea, stomach pain, heartburn, nausea, and peptic ulcers (nonhealing defects in the stomach or small intestine) as well as muscle cramps. Some people may experience side effects with one bisphosphonate, but they are able to tolerate another. Generally, less frequent dosing may lead to fewer gastrointestinal side effects.

To improve the absorption of oral bisphosphonates and to reduce the risk of gastrointestinal and esophageal side effects, it is important to follow the directions for use. First, the drug should be taken immediately after getting up in the morning, at least half an hour before eating or drinking anything besides water (even tea, coffee, fruit juice, or mineral water can interfere with absorption), and before taking any other medication. Drink at least 8 oz of water when taking the tablet, and sit or stand upright for at least 30 minutes afterward.

If you dislike taking Fosamax or Actonel every day, discuss less frequent treatment regimens with your doctor. Once-weekly regimens (70 mg of Fosamax or 35 mg of Actonel) appear to be just as effective as conventional daily dosing, and the once-weekly routine may minimize the risk of esophageal irritation. Actonel is also now available in a 150-mg tablet that can be taken monthly. Boniva can be taken orally just once a month; however, evidence of protection against hip fracture is lacking.

If you cannot tolerate oral forms of bisphosphonates because of gastrointestinal side effects, two intravenous (I.V.) forms are available: I.V. Boniva, which is given every three months, and I.V. Reclast, which is given once a year.

Another I.V. bisphosphonate is pamidronate (Aredia). Although this drug has not been approved by the FDA for the treatment of osteoporosis and limited data on fracture reduction have been published, it has been shown to improve bone mass.

Recent reports have linked bisphosphonates to osteonecrosis of the jaw (ONJ), a condition that is manifest by exposed areas of jawbone in the mouth. Invasive procedures, such as dental extraction, can increase the risk of ONJ. This condition is very rare (about 1 in 100,000 for oral bisphosphonate users), and most reported cases have been in people taking I.V. bisphosphonates in high doses for the prevention and treatment of bone metastases.

Some dentists recommend discontinuing use of these drugs for several months before and after a tooth extraction or implant surgery. Evidence to support this advice is limited but studies are ongoing. For now, it's wise to get regular dental checkups and to inform the dentist if you're taking a bisphosphonate.

Selective estrogen receptor modulators

Raloxifene (Evista) is a member of a class of drugs called selective estrogen receptor modulators (SERMs), which articles in the popular press sometimes call "designer estrogens." SERMs mimic some, but not all, of the actions of estrogen while apparently providing the

NEW RESEARCH

Sticking With Medication Reduces Fracture Risk

Women with osteoporosis would have fewer fractures if they didn't miss doses of their bisphosphonate therapy or stop taking it altogether, a new study suggests.

Researchers constructed a simulation model to assess the effect of bisphosphonate therapy on fracture rates in American women over 50 with osteoporosis. Treatment involved either daily or weekly alendronate (Fosamax) or risedronate (Actonel). The model simulated two scenarios for adherence with bisphosphonates: "optimal" adherence (defined as 90% compliance or better and no discontinuation) or "usual" adherence (defined as the current state of adherence in the United States).

As estimated by the simulation model, boosting adherence from "usual" to "optimal" would prevent 258 lifetime fractures per 1,000 women—a 23% reduction. The additional medication would cost an average of $3,800 per woman, but would save an average of $2,100 per woman in fracture-related costs—making it a low-cost way (just $1,700 over each woman's lifetime) to reduce fractures.

Side effects, cost, inconvenience, and simply forgetting all can get in the way of taking your medication. But as this study points out, skipping doses means a greater risk of broken bones.

JOURNAL OF BONE AND MINERAL RESEARCH
Published online
May 6, 2009

Drugs To Treat Osteoporosis 2010

Drug type: Brand (generic)	Typical dosages*	How to take	How they work
Bisphosphonates			
Actonel (risedronate)	5 mg/day, 35 mg 1x/week, 75 mg on 2 consecutive days each month, or 150 mg 1x/month	*Actonel and Fosamax*: Swallow whole with a full glass of water (not mineral water) at least 30 minutes before breakfast. Don't eat or drink anything but water and remain upright (sitting or standing) for 30-60 minutes. Don't take with other medications.	*Actonel, Boniva, Fosamax, and Reclast*: Reduce fracture risk by inhibiting cells that break down bone tissue (osteoclasts) and helping preserve bone mass. Vitamin D in Fosamax plus D promotes calcium absorption.
Actonel plus calcium	35 mg 1x/week plus 500 mg elemental calcium 6x/week		
Boniva (ibandronate) Intravenous Boniva (ibandronate)	2.5 mg/day or 150 mg 1x/month 3 mg 1x/3 months	*Oral Boniva only:* Wait 60 minutes after taking before consuming food, more water, or other medications. *Intravenous Boniva:* 15- to 30-second injection into a vein.	
Fosamax (alendronate)	10 mg/day or 70 mg 1x/week		
Fosamax plus D (alendronate/vitamin D)	70 mg plus 2,800 or 5,600 IU vitamin D/week		
Reclast (zoledronic acid)	5 mg 1x/year	*Reclast*: Administered intravenously over at least 15 minutes. On the day of treatment, eat and drink normally, which includes drinking at least 2 glasses of fluid, such as water, within a few hours of the infusion as directed by your doctor.	
Selective estrogen receptor modulator (SERM)			
Evista (raloxifene)	60 mg/day	Take any time with or without food.	Like HRT, replaces estrogen no longer produced by the ovaries. Acts selectively at the bone but not in the breast and uterus.
Recombinant human parathyroid hormone			
Forteo (teriparatide)	20-mcg injection 1x/day	Subcutaneous injection into thigh or abdomen.	Stimulates new bone formation, leading to increased bone mineral density and reduced risk of fractures.
Hormonal bone resorption inhibitors			
Fortical, Miacalcin (calcitonin-salmon)	200-IU spray 1x/day	Alternate nostrils daily.	Inhibits bone resorption and preserves bone mass.
Miacalcin IV (calcitonin-salmon)	200-IU injection 1x/day	Subcutaneous injection into thigh or abdomen.	

* These dosages represent an average range for the prevention or treatment of osteoporosis. The precise effective dosage varies from person to person and depends on many factors. Do not make any change in your medication without consulting your doctor.

HRT = hormone replacement therapy; NSAID = nonsteroidal anti-inflammatory drug.

Precautions	Most common side effects	Call your doctor if...
Actonel, Boniva, and Fosamax: Tell your doctor if you have kidney problems or a history of stomach problems or are taking NSAIDs or aspirin. Prevent esophagitis by taking pill as directed at left. Can (rarely) cause osteonecrosis of the jaw. Not recommended for those with kidney insufficiency or who cannot sit upright for at least 30 minutes (except intravenous Boniva). Consult your doctor to ensure that you are getting the appropriate amount of vitamin D and calcium in your supplements and diet.	*Actonel:* flu syndrome, chest pain, diarrhea, abdominal pain, nausea, constipation, difficult urination, swelling, joint pain, headache, dizziness, rash. *Boniva:* diarrhea, arm or leg pain, upset stomach. Intravenous form may cause mild reaction at injection site. *Fosamax:* abdominal pain, flu-like symptoms.	*Actonel, Boniva, and Fosamax*: You develop chest or abdominal pain, heartburn, or difficulty swallowing, develop an exposed area on the jaw bone that fails to heal or is painful.
Reclast: You should not receive Reclast if you are already receiving Zometa. Reclast and Zometa are the same medicine. They both contain zoledronic acid. If you have severe kidney problems, you should not receive Reclast. Can (rarely) cause osteonecrosis of the jaw.	*Reclast*: Fever, flu-like symptoms, muscle and joint pain, nausea, fatigue, headache. *All bisphosphonates*: Some users have (rarely) reported severe muscle, bone, or joint pain.	*Reclast*: You experience symptoms of low blood calcium (numbness or tingling around the mouth or muscle spasms) or if you have persistent pain or a nonhealing sore of the mouth or of the jaw, or if any of the most common side effects persist.
Contraindicated in women with severe liver problems or a history of blood clots. May (rarely) cause blood clots in veins or lungs. Avoid extended immobility. Should not be used along with HRT.	Hot flashes, leg cramps.	You have a history of stroke or have stroke risk factors. You develop leg pain; swelling of hands, feet, or legs; redness; chest pain; shortness of breath; vision problems; hot flashes.
Use for more than 2 years is not advised. May predispose people to digitalis toxicity. Has caused cancer in rats. Not to be used in people with a history of skeletal radiation, cancer metastasis to bone, or Paget's disease.	Nausea, dizziness, leg cramps, gout, mild reactions at injection site.	You are taking digitalis, you have had bone cancer, bone radiation, Paget's disease, or high blood calcium, you develop nausea, vomiting, constipation, lethargy, muscle weakness.
Fortical: After 30 doses, spray bottle may not deliver accurately.	*Miacalcin:* nausea, flushing, redness at injection site. *Fortical:* nasal irritation or dryness, back pain.	You develop skin rash, hives, swelling of face or throat.

continued on the next page

Drugs To Treat Osteoporosis 2010 (continued)

Drug type: Brand (generic)	Typical daily dosages*	How to take	How they work
HRT for women			
Activella (estradiol/ norethindrone acetate)	1 tablet (1 mg/0.5 mg)/day	Continuously; do not skip a week.	Replaces the estrogen no longer produced by the ovaries in postmenopausal women, thereby preserving bone mass.
Cenestin, Premarin (estrogen, conjugated)	0.3-1.25 mg/day	Continuously or 25 days on, 5 days off, as prescribed.	
Estratest, Estratest HS estrogen, esterified/ methyltestosterone)	1 tablet (1.25 mg/2.5 mg)/day; HS form: 1 tablet (0.625/1.25 mg)/day	Daily for 3 weeks, then no tablets for 1 week.	
Estrace (estradiol)	0.5-2 mg/day	23 days on, 5 days off.	
Premphase (estrogen, conjugated/ estrogen, conjugated + medroxyprogesterone)	0.625 mg/day estrogen; 0.625 mg estrogen/5 mg medroxyprogesterone 1x/day	Estrogen pill for 14 days, then combined pill for 14 days.	
Prempro (estrogen, conjugated/ medroxyprogesterone)	0.3 mg/1.5 mg; 0.45 mg /1.5 mg 0.625 mg/2.5 mg 0.625 mg/5 mg	One pill daily.	
Alora Climara Estraderm Menostar Vivelle (transdermal estradiol)	0.75-3.0 mg 2x/week 2.0-7.6 mg/week 0.05-0.1 mg 2x/week 1 mg/week 2.19-8.66 mg 2x/week	Apply patch to abdomen, buttock, or hip. Use continuously if you have had a hysterectomy; 3 weeks on, 1 week off if you have a uterus.	
Climara Pro (transdermal estradiol/levonorgestrel)	0.45 mg/d	Apply patch to abdomen. A new patch should be applied weekly during a 28-day cycle.	Same as above plus levonorgestrel reduces the risk of endometrial cancer in women with a uterus.
HRT for men			
Androderm (testosterone patch)	2.5 or 5 mg/24hr	Apply one or two patches every evening between 8 P.M. and midnight to the abdomen, back, thigh, or upper arm.	May help preserve bone mass by boosting testosterone levels, which decline in aging men.
Androgel 1% (testosterone gel)	5-10 g gel/day	Apply in the morning to upper arms, shoulders, or abdomen. Do not bathe, shower, or swim for 5-6 hours after applying.	
Delatestryl, Depo-testosterone (injectable testosterone)	50-400 mg every two to four weeks	Injected intramuscularly.	
Testim 1% (testosterone gel)	5-10 g gel/day	Apply in morning to shoulders or upper arms. Do not bathe, shower, or swim for at least 2 hours after applying.	
Striant (testosterone buccal)	30-mg pellet 2x/day	Apply pellet morning and evening to the gum just above an incisor tooth. Alternate sides of the mouth with each application.	

Precautions	Most common side effects	Call your doctor if...
Estrogen products should not be used in women with a history of blood clots or stroke; cancer of the breast, uterus, or ovaries; or in women who are pregnant. May increase risk of dementia, although this association is controversial. Women who have not had a hysterectomy should consider using products with progesterone; women who have had a hysterectomy can take estrogen without progesterone. Prempro and Premphase may cause gallbladder disease. Estratest may cause hepatitis. Have mammograms yearly. Stop taking these medications before surgery to avoid blood clots. Estrogen-containing drugs should be considered for the sole purpose of osteoporosis prevention only if other medications are not an option.	Nausea, vomiting, headache, hair loss, change in sexual drive, redness or swelling of the skin, acne, vaginal bleeding, breast pain. *Prempro or Premphase:* high blood pressure, high blood sugar, depression.	You develop breast lumps, changes in your speech, chest pain, shortness of breath, pain in your legs, unusual vaginal bleeding, vomiting, dizziness or faintness, changes in vision. *Estratest:* You develop pain, tenderness, or swelling in your abdomen or ankles, yellowing of the skin, hoarseness, acne, facial hair.
Climara Pro: Should not be used by women who have had a hysterectomy or by women with a history of blood clots or stroke; cancer of the breast, uterus, or ovaries; or by women who are pregnant.	*Climara Pro:* Headache, breast pain, irregular vaginal bleeding, stomach/abdominal cramps or bloating, nausea and vomiting, hair loss.	You develop breast lumps, changes in your speech, chest pain, shortness of breath, pain in your legs, unusual vaginal bleeding, vomiting, dizziness or faintness, changes in vision.
For use by men only. Contraindicated in men who have had breast or prostate cancer. May increase the risk of prostate cancer in healthy older men and may cause fluid retention in men with liver, kidney, or heart problems. If using testosterone gel, take all precautions in the boxed warning (such as washing hands after application) to avoid exposing others, especially pregnant women and children (children have developed enlargement of the genitals and aggressive behavior from inadvertent exposure). Avoid getting in your eyes. Do not apply Testim to the abdomen. If using a patch, change sites regularly to prevent skin irritation.	*Androderm.* Burnlike blisters, pain, redness, hardness, burning, or itching at application site. *Delatestryl and Depo-testosterone.* Breast tenderness and excessive frequency and duration of penile erections.	You develop nausea, vomiting, sleep or breathing problems, ankle swelling, erections that last too long or are too frequent, or any other unusual problems while taking testosterone.

* These dosages represent an average range for the prevention or treatment of osteoporosis. The precise effective dosage varies from person to person and depends on many factors. Do not make any change in your medication without consulting your doctor.

HRT = hormone replacement therapy; NSAID = nonsteroidal anti-inflammatory drug.

beneficial effects of estrogen without some of its negative effects.

Although Evista appears to increase bone density in the spine and the hip, studies have found significant fracture reduction only in the spine. Thus, if you have osteoporosis in the hip, Evista may not be the ideal medication for you.

The FDA approved Evista for the prevention of breast cancer in postmenopausal women with osteoporosis who are at high risk for the disease. Approval was based on findings from three clinical trials comparing Evista with placebo and a fourth comparing it with tamoxifen, which was the first drug approved by the FDA for the chemoprevention of breast cancer. In the first three trials, Evista reduced the risk of invasive breast cancer by 44 to 71% compared with placebo. In the Study of Tamoxifen and Raloxifene (STAR) trial, Evista was as effective as tamoxifen for preventing breast cancer in postmenopausal women who were at high risk for it. Both drugs reduced the risk of invasive breast cancer by about 50%.

Because of its lack of estrogen-like action on breast and uterine tissue, Evista does not cause the breast tenderness and vaginal bleeding frequently seen with estrogen therapy. In addition, Evista does not increase the risk of uterine cancer when given without progesterone. An additional benefit of Evista is its estrogen-like effect of lowering "bad" low-density lipoprotein (LDL) cholesterol. Furthermore, there appears to be no increased risk of heart attack. Although studies have not shown an increased risk of stroke, the number of serious strokes associated with Evista use was greater than the number reported with placebo.

Taking Evista does have some risks. As with estrogen therapy, there is an increased risk of serious venous thromboembolic events (the blocking of a blood vessel by a particle that has broken away from a blood clot), particularly in the first four months of therapy. Unlike estrogen, Evista does not relieve menopausal symptoms. In fact, in some studies, it increased the incidence of hot flashes.

Hormonal preparations

Estrogen and calcitonin are the hormonal preparations currently used to treat osteoporosis.

Estrogen. Used alone or with progesterone, estrogen continues to play a role in osteoporosis treatment, despite concern about its side effects (see pages 62-63). If you take estrogen for osteoporosis, use the lowest possible dose that can prevent bone loss effectively.

Calcitonin. Given by injection or nasal spray, calcitonin (Fortical, Miacalcin) is a synthetic version of a hormone produced by the human thyroid gland. It improves bone density and may slow bone loss in the spine. There appears to be a modest reduction in fracture risk in the spine; however, calcitonin does not appear to protect against hip fracture. Overall, it is not as effective as the bisphosphonates, though it does have the particular benefit of relieving the pain of recent vertebral fractures. The usual dosage is an injection every day or every other day, or one puff of nasal spray daily. Although most people tolerate the nasal spray fairly well, some may develop rhinitis (nasal inflammation).

Anabolic therapy

The only "anabolic" therapy for osteoporosis is teriparatide (Forteo), a synthetic version of human parathyroid hormone. A daily subcutaneous injection of Forteo has been shown to increase BMD dramatically and to reduce fracture in the spine and hip. Forteo works differently from antiresorptive medications in that it stimulates bone formation rather than preventing bone resorption.

One troubling potential side effect of Forteo is that it increased the risk of bone cancer in rats that were injected with high doses of the medication. Although an increase in this type of cancer has not been observed in humans treated with the medication, people at increased risk for bone cancer should not use Forteo. This includes people with Paget's disease or an unexplained rise in alkaline phosphatase levels, which would show up on a standard blood test. In addition, individuals who have undergone radiation therapy targeting bone or cancer that has spread to bone should not use Forteo.

Forteo may also raise blood calcium levels, so anyone with high levels of calcium in the blood should not use it. Forteo should not be used for more than two years, and another osteoporosis medication must be used after Forteo treatment to maintain the gain in bone density.

Treatment in Men

An underlying cause of osteoporosis can be identified in about half of the men who have the disorder. The most common causes include the use of corticosteroid medications, low testosterone levels, smoking, and excessive alcohol consumption. Treatment should be tailored to the underlying cause. For example, if testosterone levels are low, testosterone replacement therapy would be the appropriate course of treatment. In the past, testosterone could only be given by injection, usually every two weeks; today, newer preparations include skin patches (Androderm), buccal delivery through application to the cheek and gum (Striant), and testosterone gel (AndroGel, Testim), which make hormone therapy far easier.

Bone medications that are approved for the treatment of osteoporosis in men include Fosamax, Actonel, and Forteo.

Preventing Future Falls

Along with bone-strengthening medications, preventing falls is a crucial component of fracture prevention in people with osteoporosis. There are a number of simple steps you can take to reduce the likelihood of falling. First, make sure that your floors are clear of any obstacles such as area rugs or extension cords. Hallways, stairwells, and bathrooms should be well lit (especially at night). Avoid walking in stocking feet and have hand rails installed along both sides of staircases to make stairs safer. Grab bars in showers and bathtubs are highly recommended.

Be sure that your eyeglasses or contact lens prescriptions are up to date. Review your medications with your doctor; some medications can increase the risk of falls by impairing balance and alertness. In some cases, lightly padded hip protectors may be recommended; these can reduce the risk of a hip fracture in the case of a fall.

Another way to reduce the risk of falls is to improve your muscle strength through resistance training and your balance through yoga or tai chi exercises. Check with a physical therapist or certified trainer to get recommendations that are appropriate and safe for you.

Treatment of Vertebral Compression Fractures

When symptoms from a vertebral fracture are severe, rest and pain medication are recommended. Over-the-counter pain relievers may be all that is needed, although applying ice to the painful area also may be helpful. If these measures do not provide enough relief, a short-term course of prescription pain relievers may be necessary. In addition, short-term use of a back brace may prevent painful movements of the spine and reduce the length of required bed rest.

In the majority of cases, the pain associated with vertebral fractures resolves over time with conservative measures. In cases that do not get better with these therapies, surgery may be required. Surgical techniques for treating vertebral compression fractures include percutaneous vertebroplasty, kyphoplasty, and spinal fusion.

Percutaneous vertebroplasty

This minimally invasive technique is used to repair vertebral compression fractures caused by osteoporosis. The procedure involves injecting a special kind of cement called polymethylmethacrylate into both sides of the fractured vertebra. The procedure is only used for people who have suffered a recent fracture that is solely responsible for their back pain. Potential complications include soft-tissue damage and nerve-root pain and compression. There is a high level of evidence that percutaneous vertebroplasty may not be any better than placebo in the short term (see "New Research" on page 37).

Kyphoplasty

Ideally, kyphoplasty should be performed within two to three months of the fracture. Using a special balloon, the recently collapsed vertebral body is expanded and then filled with cement. As with vertebroplasty, possible complications include soft-tissue damage and nerve-root pain and compression.

Spinal fusion

In this procedure, bone grafts are used to join together two or more adjacent vertebrae. Spinal fusion may be necessary when back pain does not respond to more conservative treatments or when nerve pressure or severe deformity develops.

Treatment of Hip Fractures

Hip fractures occur in the neck of the femur (thighbone), about 1 to 2 inches from the joint or in the protrusion of the femur known as the trochanter, about 3 to 4 inches from the joint. Surgery is typically required to reposition the hipbone.

Femoral neck fractures are generally repaired in one of three ways. In the procedure known as **internal fixation**, metal screws are inserted into the bone to hold it together while it heals. In **hemiarthroplasty**, the head and neck of the femur are replaced with a metal prosthesis. **Total hip replacement** involves replacing the upper femur and socket with a prosthesis.

Surgeons repair fractures in the trochanter by inserting a metal screw, called a compression hip screw, across the bone and attaching it to a metal plate that runs down the femur. Older patients are more likely to undergo hemiarthroplasty or total hip replacement. A person who is too ill to undergo surgery may instead be placed in traction to allow the fracture to heal, but traction is a last resort because staying immobile increases the risk of blood clots.

Some complications of hip fractures include infection, deep vein thrombosis (blood clotting in the deep veins of the leg), pulmonary embolism (a blood clot that travels to the lung), pneumonia,

NEW RESEARCH

Fido and Fluffy Can Cause Falls and Fractures

Fall-related injuries sent nearly eight million Americans to emergency rooms in 2006. About 1% of these injuries were related to dogs and cats, according to a new report from the United States Centers for Disease Control and Prevention (CDC).

The CDC analyzed data from the National Electronic Injury Surveillance System All Injury Program. The data encompassed pet-related injuries treated between 2001 and 2006 in the emergency departments of 66 representative hospitals across the country.

The researchers discovered that pets are indeed significant fall hazards for Americans, especially people 75 or older—and fractures are the most common diagnosis. Approximately 23,000 fractures a year were associated with dogs and 3,000 fractures a year were associated with cats during the study period. The most frequent circumstances surrounding these injuries were falling or tripping over the pet and being pushed or pulled by a dog.

Tips to reduce your risk of pet-related falls and injuries include clearing pet items from the middle of the floor, improving lighting in your home, discouraging your pet from lying next to the foot of your chair, and, if necessary, bringing your dog to obedience school.

MMWR
Volume 58, page 277
March 27, 2009

and pressure ulcers (breaks in the skin that can become infected). Many of these complications result from bed rest and inactivity after surgery. Medications for pain control can lead to disorientation and confusion. Complications become more serious with other factors, such as older age, and the presence of other health problems.

Rehabilitation after hip fracture is essential for regaining the ability to walk and live independently. Most people who lived independently before the hip fracture will require home care and assistance. About half will require canes or walkers for several months after surgery, and nearly half of this group will need a cane or walker to move around the house or outdoors for the rest of their lives.

Treatment of Other Osteoporotic Fractures

Osteoporosis can lead to a fracture at any site in the body. The most common sites after the spine and hip are the wrist, ribs, toes, and collarbone. Treatment depends on the bone that is broken and whether or not it is displaced. Some fractures (such as wrist fractures) require a cast, while others (such as toe fractures) do not. As with all osteoporosis-related fractures, treatment focuses on relieving pain, maintaining function and mobility, treating the underlying osteoporosis, and preventing future falls. ■

acupressure—Type of massage in which continuous pressure is exerted on a trigger spot for three to five minutes.

acupuncture—Traditional Chinese treatment in which thin needles are placed at specific spots along the body.

acute—Illness or symptoms that appear suddenly and have a short course.

alkaline phosphatase—Enzyme released by bone-forming cells called osteoblasts. Blood levels of the enzyme are elevated in people with Paget's disease.

analgesic—An agent that alleviates pain without causing loss of consciousness.

ankylosing spondylitis—Chronic inflammation of the facet joints and sacroiliac joints (between the sacrum and the pelvis).

annulus fibrosus—Tough, fibrous layers of tissue that cover an intervertebral disk.

balance exercise—A type of exercise that, when practiced regularly, can increase balance and help prevent falls; examples are tai chi and yoga.

biofeedback—Back pain treatment in which the person practices different relaxation methods while using electronic sensors to measure bodily functions, such as muscle tension, breathing patterns, and heart rate.

bisphosphonates—A class of drugs that help preserve bone mass by slowing bone resorption.

body mechanics—Habitual ways of moving that can affect back health.

bone mass—The amount of bone tissue in the body.

bone mineral density testing—Radiological testing to measure bone density. Testing gives accurate measurements of the amount of bone but not the actual structure or quality of bone.

bone quality—The architecture/geometry and the material properties of bone and bone tissue.

bone remodeling—Process by which old bone is resorbed and new bone is formed.

bone resorption—Breakdown of old bone.

bone scan—Imaging test that involves injecting radioactive technetium and then measuring how much radioactivity is taken up by specific areas of bone. This test can detect metastatic cancer, bony overgrowths in Paget's disease, bacterial infections of the spine, and small fractures that are not visible on x-rays.

bone spur—See osteophytes.

calcitonin—A naturally occurring hormone involved in calcium regulation and bone metabolism.

calcium carbonate/citrate—Forms of calcium used for calcium supplementation.

cauda equina—Bundle of nerve roots at the bottom of the spinal cord.

caudal epidural block—Injection of medication directly into the base of the spine.

cervical spine—Refers to the neck.

chiropractor—Healthcare professional who uses techniques such as physical manipulation and adjustment of the spine, massage, application of heat or cold, and electrical stimulation to treat back problems.

coccyx—A term for the tailbone.

collagen—A soft protein that hardens with the deposition of calcium and phosphorus; it is a main component of bone.

Colles' fracture—A common type of fracture in which the break occurs across the end of the main bone of the forearm.

compression fracture—Fracture of a vertebral body that results in loss of height or complete collapse of the vertebral body. This type of fracture usually occurs in bones weakened by osteoporosis.

computed tomography (CAT or CT) scan—Imaging technique in which the person lies on a special table while x-rays are passed through the body and sensed by a detector that rotates 360 degrees around the person. A computer combines the information into a cross-sectional picture that shows body structures and fluids, blood clots, tumors, and bones.

CT myelogram—CT scan carried out after contrast material is injected into the spinal canal; it offers good detail of bone and soft tissue.

decompression surgery—A procedure that involves enlarging the spinal canal to relieve pressure on the spinal cord.

deep vein thrombosis (DVT)—Blood clotting that occurs in the deep veins of the leg.

dietary reference intake (DRI)—Recommended daily intake of vitamins and minerals as determined by the Institute of Medicine.

disease-modifying antirheumatic drugs—Drugs that interfere with tumor necrosis factor, which contributes to inflammation.

diskectomy—Surgical treatment for a herniated disk that takes pressure off a pinched nerve by making an incision in the annulus fibrosus and removing the extruded nucleus pulposus.

disk replacement—Surgical procedure that replaces a herniated disk with an artificial one.

displacement—Movement of bone fragments from their original positions.

dowager's hump—Kyphosis in the upper back. Common in older women, it can result from disk degeneration, the collapse of vertebrae due to osteoporosis, or both.

dual energy x-ray absorptiometry (DEXA)—A test to measure bone mineral density. Two x-ray beams are directed at the spine or hip joint, and a computer calculates the amount of energy that passes through the bone.

electromyography—A test that uses electrodes to measure muscle abnormalities.

endorphins—Pain-blocking chemicals produced by the body.

facet joints—Joints formed by the interlocking of bony projections at the rear of adjacent vertebrae.

femur—Refers to the thighbone.

flexion—A forward bending of the spine.

foramina—Spaces between adjacent vertebrae.

fracture—A break in a bone caused by injury or osteoporosis.

hemiarthroplasty—An operation to repair hip fracture that involves replacing the head and neck of the femur with a prosthesis.

herniated disk—Bulging of the central part of an intervertebral disk (nucleus pulposus) through the fibrous layers of tissue (annulus fibrosus) that cover it.

hip replacement—Surgery to implant an artificial hip joint to replace a damaged hip joint. (See also total hip replacement, hemiarthroplasty, and internal fixation.)

hormone replacement therapy (HRT)—The administration of low-dose estrogen with or without progesterone to reduce the symptoms and rapid loss of bone that accompany menopause in women. Women who have had a hysterectomy do not need to take progesterone.

hyperparathyroidism—Excessive production of parathyroid hormone by the parathyroid gland; it weakens bones by promoting loss of calcium from bone.

hyperthyroidism—Excessive production of thyroid hormone that can result in osteoporosis.

intermittent claudication—Pain in the buttocks, thighs, or calves while walking. The pain, caused by impaired blood flow to the legs, stops promptly when the person rests. The pain of spinal stenosis may be confused with intermittent claudication.

internal fixation—An operation to repair a hip fracture that involves inserting metal screws into the bone to hold it together while it heals.

intervertebral disk—Flexible pad of tissue located between vertebrae that acts as a cushion during movement, preventing vertebrae from grinding against each other.

intradiskal electrothermal therapy—A minimally invasive procedure in which the nerves in the outer wall of the disk are destroyed with a heated wire.

ipriflavone—Synthetic isoflavone that may prevent or treat osteoporosis.

isoflavone—A plant compound found in soy foods that has weak estrogen-like activity.

kyphoplasty—A new technique for treating vertebral compression fractures in which the collapsed vertebra is expanded using a special balloon and filled with cement.

kyphosis—An abnormal accentuation of the usual curvature of the upper back and commonly referred to as a humpback or hunchback.

lactose intolerance—An inability to digest the naturally occurring sugars in dairy foods.

laser diskectomy—Surgical treatment for a herniated disk that uses a laser to burn out the inside of the disk; it is a less invasive alternative to diskectomy.

lumbar spine—The lower back.

magnetic resonance imaging (MRI)—A sensitive imaging technique that surrounds a person with a powerful magnet while radio waves are passed through the body.

massage therapy—A therapy used to ease tension and relax back muscles.

microdiskectomy—A surgical treatment for a herniated disk that is done through a very small opening, it is a less invasive alternative to diskectomy.

muscle relaxants—Drugs that depress the activity of nerves in the spinal cord and brain. Used with caution as they can cause drowsiness and are potentially addictive.

nerve conduction test—A test that examines nerve function.

n-telopeptides—A byproduct of the breakdown of bone that can be measured in urine tests.

nucleus pulposus—The central part of an intervertebral disk that, as a person ages, slowly loses its water content and shrinks.

open laminectomy—A surgical procedure for a herniated disk in which a small part of the vertebra is removed.

opiates—Drugs that depress the nervous system to block the perception of pain. As they are potentially addictive and have many side effects, they are used for back pain only when all other options have failed.

osteoblasts—Cells that fill small cavities in the bone surface with new bone during bone formation.

osteoclasts—Cells that invade the surface of bone and remove the matrix and minerals, leaving small cavities in the bone surface during bone resorption.

osteomalacia—A softening of bone that results from a lack of the essential minerals calcium and phosphorus.

osteopenia—Low bone mass.

osteophyte—A bony overgrowth, or spur.

osteoporosis—A disease marked by progressively decreasing bone mass; it results in weakened, brittle bones that can fracture easily.

Paget's disease—A condition characterized by excessive overgrowth of bone, especially in the spine, pelvis, skull, and femur.

palliative treatment—Therapy aimed at relieving pain and limiting disease complications rather than curing the disease.

parathyroid hormone—Hormone of the parathyroid gland that regulates calcium and phosphorus metabolism throughout the body.

pelvis—Basin-shaped structure in the lower part of the trunk composed of the two hipbones, tailbone (coccyx), and lower backbone (sacrum).

percutaneous arthroscopic diskectomy—Surgical treatment for a herniated disk that is less invasive than diskectomy; the procedure involves inserting a probe into the disk to scoop it out.

percutaneous vertebroplasty—A minimally invasive technique to treat vertebral compression fractures. Involves the injection of cement into the fractured vertebra.

perimenopause—The time immediately before menopause begins.

peripheral dual-energy x-ray absorptiometry—A bone density test that is similar to DEXA and uses a portable machine to measure bone density in the finger, wrist, or heel.

peripheral quantitative computed tomography—A bone density test that is similar to QCT (see below) and measures bone density in the wrist.

peripheral sites—Bone sites other than those central to the body (spine and hip), such as the wrist, heel, and finger.

processes—Bony projections jutting out from the rear of a vertebra.

pulmonary embolism—A blood clot that blocks one of the blood vessels in the lungs.

pyridinium cross-links—A product created by the breakdown of bone that can be measured in urine tests.

quantitative computed tomography (QCT)—A test used to determine vertebral density by measuring the absorption of radiation by bone.

quantitative ultrasound—A technique that uses sound waves to measure bone density in peripheral sites.

radiographic absorptiometry—A technique that uses x-rays to measure bone density in the hand.

relaxation therapy—Treatment that teaches techniques of muscle relaxation and breathing so that a person can deal better with stress, a possible cause of back pain.

resistance exercise—A type of exercise that entails working muscles against weights.

sacroiliac joints—Joints on either side of the sacrum that join the sacrum to the other bones of the pelvis.

sacrum—The flat, triangular bone formed by the fusion of the lowest five vertebrae.

sciatic nerve—The nerve arising from the lower spine that extends into the leg and foot.

sciatica—Pain that radiates into the buttocks, down the thighs, into the calves, and often into the feet; the pain is caused by irritation of the sciatic nerve.

scoliosis—An abnormal sideways bend to the back caused by twisting of the spine.

secondary osteoporosis—Osteoporosis caused by certain medications or other diseases.

selective estrogen receptor modulators (SERMS)—A class of drugs that mimic the actions of estrogen in some tissues and block the effects of estrogen in others.

sensory-evoked potential—A test to examine nerve function.

sequestration—A condition in which fragments of a herniated disk break free.

single-energy x-ray absorptiometry—A test used to measure bone density in the wrist or heel, similar to DEXA, except that it uses one x-ray beam.

spasm—A sudden, involuntary muscle contraction that produces pain; spasms can occur when a muscle or ligament in the back is torn or when a disk or facet joint is injured.

trochanter—Part of the femur that protrudes below the bone's neck.

ultrasound—The use of high-frequency sound waves to detect osteoporosis and predict the risk of fractures.

vertebra, vertebrae (pl.)—Any of the 33 interlocking bones that form the spinal column.

vertebral compression fracture—Collapse of the front of a vertebra, often producing immediate and intense pain in the area of the fracture; it can be caused by even minor trauma in a vertebra weakened by cancer, osteoporosis, Paget's disease, or hyperparathyroidism.

vertebral osteomyelitis—A serious bacterial infection of the spine that can cause pain in the neck or back and is usually accompanied by fever.

weight-bearing exercise—Exercise such as walking, jogging, or stair climbing, in which the bones of the feet, legs, and spine bear the body's weight.

ABBREVIATIONS AND ACRONYMS

ACR—American College of Rheumatology
BMD—bone mineral density
BSAP—bone-specific alkaline phosphatase
CAT—computerized axial tomography
CDC—Centers for Disease Control and Prevention
CT—computed tomography
CTX—C-terminal type 1 collagen telopeptide
DMARD—disease-modifying antirheumatic drug
DPD—deoxypyridinoline
DRI—dietary reference intake
DXA—dual-energy x-ray absorptiometry
FDA—U.S. Food and Drug Administration
FRAX—fracture risk assessment tool
HRT—hormone replacement therapy
I.V.—intravenous
IDET—intradiskal electrothermal therapy
LDL—low-density lipoprotein
MAO—monoamine oxidase
MRI—magnetic resonance imaging
NSAID—nonsteroidal anti-inflammatory drug
NTX—N-terminal type 1 collagen telopeptide
ONJ—osteonecrosis of the jaw
pDXA—peripheral dual-energy x-ray absorptiometry
pQCT—peripheral quantitative computed tomography
PSA—proton-specific antigen
QCT—quantitative computed tomography
QUS—quantitative ultrasound
RA—radiographic absorptiometry
SERM—selective estrogen receptor modulator
STAR—Study of Tamoxifen and Raloxifene
SXA—single-energy x-ray absorptiometry
TENS—transcutaneous electrical nerve stimulation
TRAP—tartrate-resistant acid phosphatase

HEALTH INFORMATION ORGANIZATIONS AND SUPPORT GROUPS

American Academy of Medical Acupuncture
1970 E. Grand Ave., Ste. 330
El Segundo, CA 90245
☎ 310-364-0193
www.medicalacupuncture.org
Provides referrals for physicians throughout the country who practice acupuncture. Promotes awareness, education, and integration of acupuncture concepts with Western medical training.

American Academy of Orthopaedic Surgeons
6300 N. River Rd.
Rosemont, IL 60018-4262
☎ 847-823-7186
www.aaos.org
Provides referrals to orthopedists in your area. Publishes information on orthopedic disorders.

American Osteopathic Association
142 E. Ontario St.
Chicago, IL 60611
☎ 800-621-1773/312-202-8000
www.osteopathic.org
National association of roughly 61,000 osteopathic physicians. Advances the practice and knowledge of osteopathic medicine, provides certification to osteopaths, and accredits osteopathic medical colleges and healthcare facilities.

American Pain Society
4700 W. Lake Ave.
Glenview, IL 60025
☎ 847-375-4715
www.ampainsoc.org
Provides information on pain centers throughout the country. Advances pain-related research, education, treatment, and professional practice.

Arthritis Foundation
P.O. Box 7669
Atlanta, GA 30357-0669
☎ 800-283-7800
www.arthritis.org
Provides information about causes, symptoms, diagnosis, and treatment of arthritis. Makes referrals to local chapters and offers services to improve quality of life for people with arthritis through support groups and social activities.

Commission on Accreditation of Rehabilitation Facilities
4891 E. Grant Rd.
Tucson, AZ 85712
☎ 888-281-6531/520-325-1044
www.carf.org
Nonprofit organization that provides accreditation in the human services field, focusing on the areas of rehabilitation, behavioral health, and aging services. Can provide a list of accredited rehabilitation facilities in your area.

National Certification Commission for Acupuncture and Oriental Medicine
76 South Laura St., Ste. 1290
Jacksonville, FL 32202
☎ 904-598-1005
www.nccaom.org
Establishes, assesses, and promotes standards of competence and safety for acupuncture. Provides an online directory designed for individuals seeking practitioners who meet requirements for board certification in acupuncture and other types of Asian therapy.

The National Institutes of Health Osteoporosis and Related Bone Diseases National Resource Center
2 AMS Circle
Bethesda, MD 20892-3676
☎ 800-624-2663/202-223-0344/202-466-4315 (TTY)
www.niams.nih.gov/bone
Provides information on diseases of the bone, including osteoporosis, Paget's disease, osteogenesis imperfecta, and hyperparathyroidism.

National Osteoporosis Foundation
1232 22nd St. NW
Washington, DC 20037-1202
☎ 800-231-4222/202-223-2226
www.nof.org
National volunteer health agency dedicated to reducing the prevalence of osteoporosis and promoting bone health. Information on osteoporosis prevention and treatment is available online or by request.

LEADING HOSPITALS
for Orthopedics as Ranked by *U.S. News & World Report*

1. **Mayo Clinic**
   Rochester, MN
   ☎ 507-284-2511
   www.mayoclinic.org

2. **Hospital for Special Surgery**
   New York, NY
   ☎ 212-606-1000
   www.hss.edu

3. **Massachusetts General Hospital**
   Boston, MA
   ☎ 617-726-2000
   www.massgeneral.org

4. **Cleveland Clinic**
   Cleveland, OH
   ☎ 216-444-2200
   www.clevelandclinic.org

5. **Johns Hopkins Hospital**
   Baltimore, MD
   ☎ 410-955-5000
   www.hopkinsmedicine.org

6. **Duke University Medical Center**
   Durham, NC
   ☎ 919-684-8111
   www.dukehealth.org

7. **New York-Presbyterian University Hospital of Columbia and Cornell**
   New York, NY
   ☎ 212-746-5454
   www.nyp.org

8. **University of Iowa Hospitals and Clinics**
   Iowa City, IA
   ☎ 319-356-1616
   www.uihealthcare.com

9. **New York University Hospital for Joint Diseases**
   New York, NY
   ☎ 212-263-7300
   www.nyumedicalcenter.org

10. **University of Pittsburgh Medical Center**
    Pittsburgh, PA
    ☎ 412-647-2345
    www.upmc.com

INDEX

NOTES

NOTES

The information contained in this White Paper is not intended as a substitute for the advice of a physician. Readers who suspect they may have specific medical problems should consult a physician about any suggestions made.

Please address inquiries on bulk subscriptions and permission to reproduce selections from this White Paper to The Johns Hopkins White Papers, MediZine LLC, 500 Fifth Avenue, Suite 1900, New York, NY 10110.

The editors are interested in receiving your comments at whitepapers@johnshopkinshealthalerts.com or the above address but regret that they cannot answer letters of any sort personally.

ISBN 978-1-935584-01-8

Printed in the United States of America

JOHNS HOPKINS
MEDICINE

The Johns Hopkins White Papers are produced by University Health Publishing, a division of MediZine LLC.

2010 WHITE PAPER TITLES

ARTHRITIS 2010 - Covers the three most common forms of arthritis—osteoarthritis, rheumatoid arthritis, and gout—as well as two other rheumatic diseases: fibromyalgia and bursitis.

BACK PAIN and OSTEOPOROSIS 2010 - Addresses back pain due to sprains, strains, and spasms; degenerative changes of the spinal bones and disks; disk herniation; and spinal stenosis. Also covers osteoporosis, a common cause of fractures in the spine and hip.

COLON CANCER 2010 - Explains how colorectal cancer begins and discusses screening, diagnosis, and treatment options for colon cancer, rectal cancer, and metastasized cancer. Special charts review common chemotherapy drugs, regimens, and staging systems for colorectal cancer.

CORONARY HEART DISEASE 2010 - Discusses four problems resulting from coronary heart disease: angina, heart attacks, heart failure, and arrhythmias.

DEPRESSION and ANXIETY 2010 - Includes major depression, dysthymia, atypical depression, bipolar disorder, seasonal affective disorder, panic disorder, generalized anxiety disorder, obsessive-compulsive disorder, post-traumatic stress disorder, and phobic disorders.

DIABETES 2010 - Shows you how to manage your diabetes and avoid complications such as foot problems and vision changes. Reviews the latest tools for monitoring your blood glucose and the newest medications for controlling it.

DIGESTIVE DISORDERS 2010 - Covers gastroesophageal reflux disease, peptic ulcers, dysphagia, achalasia, Barrett's esophagus, esophageal spasm and stricture, gastritis, gallstones, diarrhea, celiac disease, constipation, Crohn's disease, ulcerative colitis, and colon cancer.

HEART ATTACK PREVENTION 2010 - Provides up-to-date strategies for preventing a first heart attack, including identifying possible risk factors, the latest screening tests, risk-reducing lifestyle measures, and medications for controlling cholesterol.

HYPERTENSION and STROKE 2010 - Explains how to treat your high blood pressure and prevent it from harming your health. Also covers the two forms of stroke: ischemic stroke and hemorrhagic stroke.

LUNG DISORDERS 2010 - Includes information on emphysema and chronic bronchitis (together referred to as chronic obstructive pulmonary disease, or COPD), asthma, pneumonia, lung cancer, and sleep apnea.

MEMORY 2010 - Tells you how to keep your memory sharp as you get older and how to recognize the symptoms of age-associated memory impairment, mild cognitive impairment, and illnesses such as Alzheimer's disease and vascular dementia.

NUTRITION and WEIGHT CONTROL for LONGEVITY 2010 - Gives you the information you need to eat a healthy diet and keep your weight under control. Also explains what to do when the pounds just don't seem to budge.

PRESCRIPTION DRUGS 2010 - Discusses drug development and the FDA approval process, drug delivery systems, off-label prescribing, and advice on generic drug safety, drug side effects, adherence issues, and much more.

PROSTATE DISORDERS 2010 - Helps you decide among the various treatment options for prostate cancer, benign prostatic hyperplasia, and prostatitis.

VISION 2010 - Reviews the current knowledge on cataracts, glaucoma, age-related macular degeneration, and diabetic retinopathy. Also discusses ways to cope with low vision.

60ABWP

The 2010 White Papers

Take Control of Your Medical Condition

JOHNS HOPKINS MEDICINE

Visit us online at www.JohnsHopkinsHealthAlerts.com/bookstore

YES, I've placed a check mark next to the White Paper(s) I'd like to receive for $19.95 each. Annual updates on each subject that I have chosen will be offered to me by announcement card. I need do nothing if I want the update to be sent to me automatically. If I do not want it, I will return the announcement card marked "cancel." I may cancel at any time. (Please add $2.95 for domestic, $4.95 for Canadian, and $15.00 for foreign orders to your total to cover shipping and handling.) (CT, FL, IL, MA and OH residents add sales tax.)

✔ Please put a check mark next to the White Paper(s) you wish to order.

001107	❑ Arthritis	$19.95	008102	❑ Prostate Disorders	$19.95
003103	❑ Coronary Heart Disease	$19.95	010108	❑ Digestive Disorders	$19.95
004101	❑ Depression and Anxiety	$19.95	011106	❑ Vision	$19.95
005108	❑ Diabetes	$19.95	012104	❑ Back Pain & Osteoporosis	$19.95
006106	❑ Hypertension and Stroke	$19.95	015107	❑ Memory	$19.95
007104	❑ Nutrition and Weight Control for Longevity	$19.95	019109	❑ Lung Disorders	$19.95
			020107	❑ Heart Attack Prevention	$19.95
021601	Prescription Drugs (online only)	$19.95	022609	Colon Cancer (online only)	$19.95

Name

Address

City State Zip

METHOD OF PAYMENT: (U.S. funds only) ❑ VISA ❑ MasterCard ❑ Check Enclosed ❑ Bill Me

Credit Card # Exp. Date

Signature Date

Money Back Guarantee: If for any reason, you are not satisfied after receipt of your publications, return your purchase within 30 days for a full refund.

Detach and mail this card back to The Johns Hopkins White Papers, P.O. Box 420083, Palm Coast, FL 32142

60ABWP

The 2010 White Papers

Take Control of Your Medical Condition

JOHNS HOPKINS MEDICINE

Visit us online at www.JohnsHopkinsHealthAlerts.com/bookstore

YES, I've placed a check mark next to the White Paper(s) I'd like to receive for $19.95 each. Annual updates on each subject that I have chosen will be offered to me by announcement card. I need do nothing if I want the update to be sent to me automatically. If I do not want it, I will return the announcement card marked "cancel." I may cancel at any time. (Please add $2.95 for domestic, $4.95 for Canadian, and $15.00 for foreign orders to your total to cover shipping and handling.) (CT, FL, IL, MA and OH residents add sales tax.)

✔ Please put a check mark next to the White Paper(s) you wish to order.

001107	❑ Arthritis	$19.95	008102	❑ Prostate Disorders	$19.95
003103	❑ Coronary Heart Disease	$19.95	010108	❑ Digestive Disorders	$19.95
004101	❑ Depression and Anxiety	$19.95	011106	❑ Vision	$19.95
005108	❑ Diabetes	$19.95	012104	❑ Back Pain & Osteoporosis	$19.95
006106	❑ Hypertension and Stroke	$19.95	015107	❑ Memory	$19.95
007104	❑ Nutrition and Weight Control for Longevity	$19.95	019109	❑ Lung Disorders	$19.95
			020107	❑ Heart Attack Prevention	$19.95
021601	Prescription Drugs (online only)	$19.95	022609	Colon Cancer (online only)	$19.95

Name

Address

City State Zip

METHOD OF PAYMENT: (U.S. funds only) ❑ VISA ❑ MasterCard ❑ Check Enclosed ❑ Bill Me

Credit Card # Exp. Date

Signature Date

Money Back Guarantee: If for any reason, you are not satisfied after receipt of your publications, return your purchase within 30 days for a full refund.

Detach and mail this card back to The Johns Hopkins White Papers, P.O. Box 420083, Palm Coast, FL 32142

Cut on dotted line

Johns Hopkins White Papers

Fold along this line and tape closed

NO POSTAGE
NECESSARY
IF MAILED
IN THE
UNITED STATES

BUSINESS REPLY MAIL

FIRST-CLASS MAIL PERMIT NO. 86 FLAGLER BEACH FL

POSTAGE WILL BE PAID BY ADDRESSEE

THE JOHNS HOPKINS WHITE PAPERS
PO BOX 420083
PALM COAST FL 32142-9966

Johns Hopkins White Papers

Fold along this line and tape closed

NO POSTAGE
NECESSARY
IF MAILED
IN THE
UNITED STATES

BUSINESS REPLY MAIL

FIRST-CLASS MAIL PERMIT NO. 86 FLAGLER BEACH FL

POSTAGE WILL BE PAID BY ADDRESSEE

THE JOHNS HOPKINS WHITE PAPERS
PO BOX 420083
PALM COAST FL 32142-9966